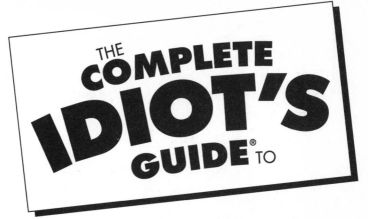

# Reflexology

D0965223

## Second Edition

*by Frankie Avalon Wolfe, Ph.D.*

ALPHA

A member of Penguin Group (USA) Inc.

## ALPHA BOOKS

Published by the Penguin Group

Penguin Group (USA) Inc., 375 Hudson Street, New York, New York 10014, U.S.A.

Penguin Group (Canada), 10 Alcorn Avenue, Toronto, Ontario, Canada M4V 3B2 (a division of Pearson Penguin Canada Inc.)

Penguin Books Ltd, 80 Strand, London WC2R 0RL, England

Penguin Ireland, 25 St Stephen's Green, Dublin 2, Ireland (a division of Penguin Books Ltd)

Penguin Group (Australia), 250 Camberwell Road, Camberwell, Victoria 3124, Australia (a division of Pearson Australia Group Pty Ltd)

Penguin Books India Pvt Ltd, 11 Community Centre, Panchsheel Park, New Delhi—10 017, India

Penguin Group (NZ), cnr Airborne and Rosedale Roads, Albany, Auckland 1310, New Zealand (a division of Pearson New Zealand Ltd)

Penguin Books (South Africa) (Pty) Ltd, 24 Sturdee Avenue, Rosebank, Johannesburg 2196, South Africa

Penguin Books Ltd, Registered Offices: 80 Strand, London WC2R 0RL, England

## Copyright © 2006 by Frankie Avalon Wolfe, Ph.D.

International Standard Book Number: 1-59257-529-3
Library of Congress Catalog Card Number: 2006920727

08    07    06        8    7    6    5    4    3    2    1

Interpretation of the printing code: The rightmost number of the first series of numbers is the year of the book's printing; the rightmost number of the second series of numbers is the number of the book's printing. For example, a printing code of 06-1 shows that the first printing occurred in 2006.

*Printed in the United States of America*

**Note:** This publication contains the opinions and ideas of its author. It is intended to provide helpful and informative material on the subject matter covered. It is sold with the understanding that the author and publisher are not engaged in rendering professional services in the book. If the reader requires personal assistance or advice, a competent professional should be consulted.

The author and publisher specifically disclaim any responsibility for any liability, loss, or risk, personal or otherwise, which is incurred as a consequence, directly or indirectly, of the use and application of any of the contents of this book.

Most Alpha books are available at special quantity discounts for bulk purchases for sales promotions, premiums, fundraising, or educational use. Special books, or book excerpts, can also be created to fit specific needs.

For details, write: Special Markets, Alpha Books, 375 Hudson Street, New York, NY 10014.

**Publisher:** *Marie Butler-Knight*
**Editorial Director:** *Mike Sanders*
**Managing Editor:** *Billy Fields*
**Senior Acquisitions Editor:** *Randy Ladenheim-Gil*
**Development Editor:** *Christy Wagner*
**Senior Production Editor:** *Janette Lynn*

**Copy Editor:** *Tricia Liebig*
**Book Designers:** *Trina Wurst/Kurt Owens*
**Cover Designer:** *Rebecca Harmon*
**Indexer:** *Tonya Heard*
**Layout:** *Brian Massey*
**Proofreader:** *John Etchison*

# Contents at a Glance

WITHDRAWN

# Contents

# Foreword

Reflexology is an ancient healing art that came to us from China, Egypt, and India and was rediscovered more than 100 years ago. Like other ancient healing modalities, we have been able to rediscover reflexology's many benefits, and we are able to use these benefits to assist us in alleviating the stresses of the modern world.

Reflexology has the ability to bring about a state of relaxation, and because of this, it is able to assist the body's own natural healing to take place. Reflexology is also able to complement other types of health care. From my own experiences, I have found that reflexology is able to assist everyone, from infants right through to the elderly. It is of benefit whether our lives take active or sedentary roles, and it is able to transcend all barriers: emotional, physical, and mental.

With the increased interest in reflexology worldwide, I find it exciting that the amount of information available to the general public on this subject is increasing. It is refreshing to see a book like *The Complete Idiot's Guide to Reflexology* being published, especially this updated and revised second edition. This book explains the workings of reflexology to the layperson in easy-to-understand terms and still manages to contain a wealth of information for the complete novice.

It covers all the body systems and explains in simple terms the importance of each system. It covers everything the beginner needs to know and might come across when giving sessions to family and friends. It also tells you the different types of foot conditions that can occur and the importance of wearing the correct shoes.

It has been said that the foot is a reflection of our health, and reflexology gives us a means to use this reflection to improve the health of our family and friends. I hope that you will find *The Complete Idiot's Guide to Reflexology, Second Edition*, to be of great benefit.

Russell McAllister

Russell McAllister is publisher of *Reflexology World* magazine and a director of the International Council of Reflexologists. Mr. McAllister is a founding member of the Reflexology Association of Australia and resides in Sydney, Australia, where he has a reflexology practice.

# Introduction

When I was first asked to write this book, I was delighted—and then immediately anxious. I thought, *How can I write a nearly 300-page book on the basics of reflexology and keep it entertaining?*

I thought about how over the years I have been helped by reflexology and how my clients have responded to their treatments. I thought about how reflexology is more than just a therapy involving pushing reflex points, but is also a philosophy. It shows us how our body is connected and how it reacts to stimulus and mirrors how the world is connected. This connection idea is a philosophical point of view I use in my life and my practice.

I decided to include some "fun" ideas you might find useful, such as how to read the personality in the feet. We all have the personal power to behave correctly; however, it's entertaining to match the general personality tendencies with the shape and condition of a foot. This observance is not necessarily considered part of reflexology, but because you'll be observing feet, you might be surprised how many times the foot fits the person! Utilizing this technique, you may be able to understand a little more about a person and help personalize how you deal with them.

I hope you have fun reading this book and that you laugh, learn, and grow. I wish you the best of health.

## How to Use This Book

The book is divided into four parts:

**Part 1, "Before You Take Off Your Socks,"** introduces you to the theory of reflexology, what it means, and what it's used for.

**Part 2, "Tools and Techniques for Feeling Good,"** gets into the proper techniques of reflexology to help you focus on getting results.

**Part 3, "The Body Systems: Mapping It Out,"** covers all the body systems and describes where the major reflex points are mapped on the feet and hands.

Part 4, "Out of Step: Identifying (and Avoiding) Foot Problems," gives you some insight into the physical conditions of the foot. It also helps you see how your feet can tell a story about you.

## Extras

In addition to all the things you'll learn in the text, this book has some special features to make your progress even more pleasant. Let me introduce you to a few extras you'll see in this book:

---

### def•i•ni•tion

These boxes highlight the terminology used in reflexology and give you the language you need to describe what you're doing.

---

### Foot Note

These boxes contain anecdotal information, personal stories, and extra bits of information about reflexology. Read them to find out a little bit more.

---

### Tread Lightly

These boxes warn you about things you need to be cautious about. They include warnings, contraindications, and important pointers to things you need to take seriously.

---

### Tip Toe

These boxes contain little tidbits of information and highlight important facts about reflexology. Some include tips that help you do things more easily.

---

## Acknowledgments

I've been humbled by the vast amounts of fan mail readers have sent me from around the world since the release of the first edition of this book. Hearing how my books have helped you directly and even inspired some of you to make career changes touches me deeply. So the first note of appreciation must go to my readers. It is because of those of you who enjoy learning and laughing that these books are available and that a second edition of this book was created. And thank you Alpha Books, for including me as an author for such a great series.

I owe a great deal of gratitude to those at Alpha Books who put so much work into this abridged and updated second edition. You've all made it possible for this release despite my overwhelming distractions from the many aspects of my business and personal events. It simply wouldn't have been possible without such a great team.

Specifically, thank you Randy Ladenheim-Gil for being so positive and guiding the initiation of this project, and of course thank you Marie Butler-Knight for the generous opportunity to give new life to the old version. And my thanks especially to Shelly Hager, who did so much work cutting away material from the original version and patching it back up to maintain the flow while still keeping the essentials that the readers want to know about reflexology. Thank you Tricia Liebig for your editing assistance. And of course Christy Wagner, who, although you cut out a lot of my silly jokes, are a definite pro and a delight to work with; thanks for reining in my diversions.

And as always, no one writes a book or works on a big project (happily at least) without the support and encouragement of their loved ones. I've had the gift of patience from my husband and close family and friends of not complaining about being neglected while I obsessively work on a project. To you I say, I can't promise I'll be less obsessive, but I can promise that my next obsessive goal will be to work on balancing my work and social life! And thank you to all my clients, who over the years have proven just how positively transforming a natural health lifestyle can be.

## Special Thanks to the Technical Reviewer

*The Complete Idiot's Guide to Reflexology, Second Edition*, was reviewed by an M.D. expert who double-checked the medical accuracy of what you'll learn here.

## Trademarks

All terms mentioned in this book that are known to be or are suspected of being trademarks or service marks have been appropriately capitalized. Alpha Books and Penguin Group (USA) Inc. cannot attest to the accuracy of this information. Use of a term in this book should not be regarded as affecting the validity of any trademark or service mark.

# Before You Take Off Your Socks

Before you expose your toes, we need to cover some reflexology basics! Reflexology is a natural, safe, and effective practice that helps you take responsibility for your health. Reflexology can be used in three different ways, which is one reason it is so much fun to learn.

First of all, reflexology is primarily used as a natural therapy to promote relaxation and healing of the body, mind, and soul. Secondly, you can use reflexology as part of a health analysis, because your feet and hands give clues about what is going on inside your body. And finally, you can use the clues observed on your feet and hands as a tool for discovering your hidden personality traits.

In Part 1, we take a stroll through the basics of reflexology and the fundamental structure and makeup of the feet. Let's go!

# Chapter 1

# What Is Reflexology?

## In This Chapter

- Understand what reflexology is
- Learn how reflexology works
- Discover how to think holistically
- Realize the different uses of reflexology
- See how reflexology complements other holistic therapies

When I heard that my friend, who was working as a pedicurist, was taking a class in reflexology, I immediately jumped at the chance to join her. I had no clue what reflexology was all about, but I did know it had something to do with natural healing. When we began working on each other as students, I felt like my entire insides had been toned and refreshed! The cold that I was beginning to get the day before class had spontaneously disappeared, and the bladder infection I felt coming on went away!

These results all came within the first 4 hours of my first class, and I knew that I was passionately interested in learning more about the natural, ancient, safe, and effective healing therapy known as reflexology.

This chapter leads you feet first through the philosophy behind reflexology, how it works, and how simply it can fit into your life.

# Reflexology: Go with the Flow

Let's start by going over the basic definition of reflexology so we can get to the good stuff quickly! Broken down into its basic parts, the word *reflexology* is made up of *reflex*, in this case meaning one part reflecting another part, and *ology*, meaning the study of. Put together, reflexology means the study of how one part relates to another part. But fortunately for those of us who love to get and give reflexology sessions, there's much more to it than just the study of its parts!

**def•i•ni•tion**

**Reflexology** literally means the study of how one part of the body reflects or relates to another part. It's a holistic therapy used for health management and maintenance and can also be used as a health- and personality-analysis tool.

Reflexology is commonly explained as the scientific theory that maps out the reflexes on the feet and hands to all the organs and the rest of the body. In other words, certain spots on the feet and hands have an energy connection to other parts of your body. By applying acupressure and massagelike techniques to the feet and hands, you can positively affect all other body parts.

Although they share some similarities, acupressure, massage, and reflexology are all distinctly separate therapies from each other. (For a description of acupressure and acupuncture, see the appendix) Also, don't confuse reflexology with massage—it goes much deeper than that!

Throughout this book I refer to *reflexes* or *reflex points*, *areas*, or *spots*. These all mean the same thing. A reflex area or spot is a spot on the hands, feet, or ears that corresponds to a body part or organ elsewhere on the body. For instance, if I indicate to "Press on your kidney reflex," I'm describing where on your feet or hands the corresponding reflex points for the kidneys are. By applying pressure in these areas, you can positively affect your kidney(s). The following figures show the reflex points on the hands and the feet.

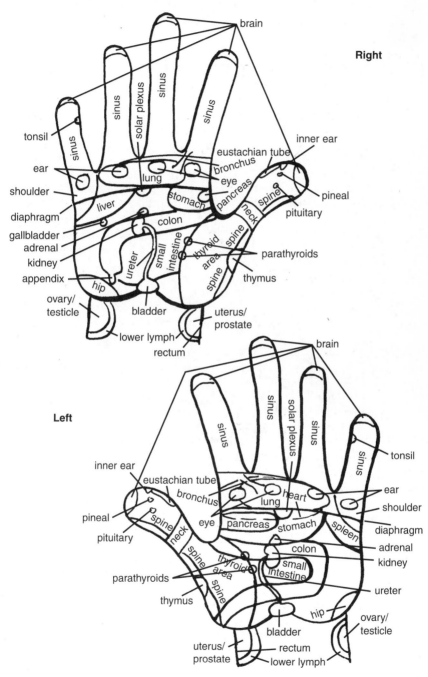

*The reflex points on the hands.*

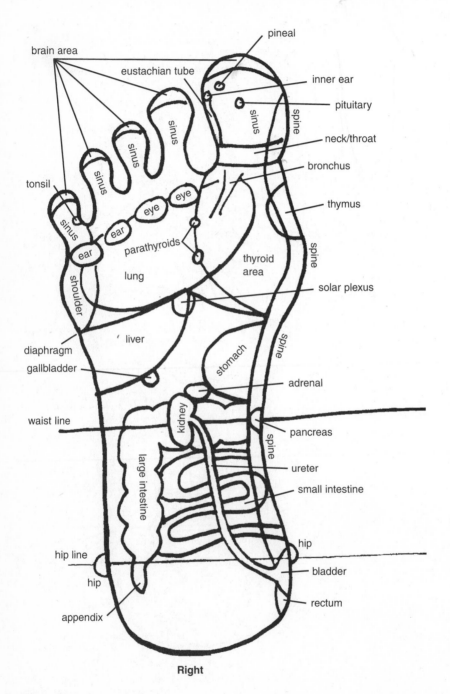

*The reflex points on the feet.*

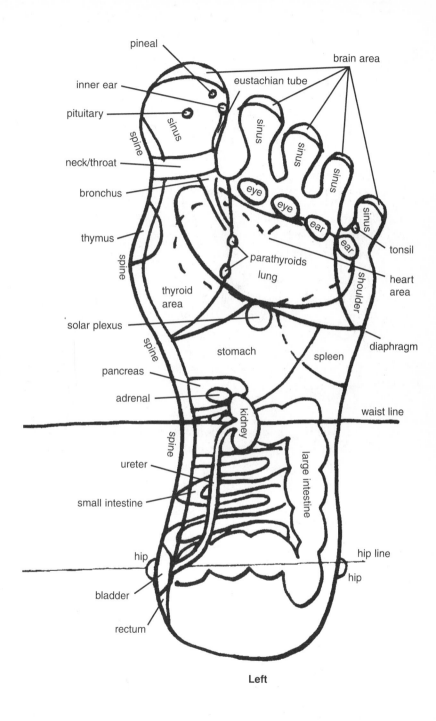

**Left**

## Fancy Footwork

Reflexology is more than just the study of reflex points. It's also a wonderful, natural health therapy; a health-analysis tool; and sometimes it's even used to reveal the personality of the foot owner! Locating the places on the feet that correspond to different areas is great, but the true beauty of reflexology is what you can learn about yourself or your partner when you practice reflexology on them. Of course, another beauty of reflexology is how good it makes you feel!

Reflexology can be used in three ways:

- ◆ **As a hands-on natural health body therapy.** The feet, hands, and sometimes ears are worked on to create relaxation, ease pain, and stimulate the body's ability to heal itself.

- ◆ **As a health-analysis tool.** Medical doctors are the only practitioners allowed to diagnose diseases; however, when performing reflexology, you'll recognize many types of foot ailments, which will give you the opportunity to get proper treatment. Also, by finding tender reflex spots in your own feet or hands, you just might be able to discern something about the condition of the corresponding organ. (See Chapters 17 and 18 for more on these subjects.)

- ◆ **As a personality-analysis tool.** Some practitioners can discern things about the recipient's personality by observing the shapes, lines, and conditions of their feet and hands. Although this isn't technically considered within the scope of reflexology, it's harmless fun and can be surprisingly accurate! (See Chapter 19 for more information.)

## The Whole Story

Because the body works as a whole unit, reflex points can actually be found in many places in the body. In other words, your body is all connected; you cannot isolate any one part of the body completely without it ceasing to function. The holistic practitioner understands this "whole" concept and utilizes this knowledge to create natural therapies that apply to the whole body. Several practices map out reflex areas:

- **Foot, hand, and ear reflexology.** That's what this book is all about! However, in this book, I primarily concentrate on the reflexes on the feet.

- **Bowel reflexes.** Natural health practitioners also believe the bowel has reflex points in it. This means that an irritation or pain experienced in some part of the body may be linked to stagnation or some type of problem found in the bowel.

- **Iris reflexes or iridology.** This fascinating study is based on the idea that the iris of the eye (the colored part) reflects inherent weaknesses or tendencies within the body—kind of like how a computer screen or a TV projects an image. The iris is divided into pie-shaped pieces that map out the entire body. A trained iridologist utilizes the iris map and "reads your eyes," your genetic makeup, and other information about your body.

- **Body reflexology.** Mildred Carter, famous for her foot and hand reflexology work, also has made body reflexology quite popular. Basically, the system maps out reflex points located in various areas on the body (even the tongue) that when pressed affect a different area of the body.

You cannot isolate one area of your body and only affect that area. In fact, whatever you're exposed to or ingest has some effect on every part of you. If you take very good care of at least one part of you, all the other parts benefit. So in this book, I keep it simple and fun and concentrate on taking very good care of our feet. Just keep in mind that, like everything in life, the whole is always greater than the sum of its parts!

## Putting Your Foot in Your Mouth

Reflexology is not just fancy footwork. In fact, many reflexologists are adamant that you never call their practice a "foot rub" or "foot (and/or hand) massage." I tend to be more relaxed about semantics, but sometimes these terms can get you in trouble. I learned this embarrassing lesson years ago when I was taking my first reflexology class at The Colorado School of Healing Arts.

**Tread Lightly** _____

Most reflexologists prefer to have you call what they do *reflexology sessions*, or *hand and foot reflexology*, not foot and hand massage or foot rubs.

I was so excited about learning this new skill that I would practically grab any poor, innocent bystander I could find just for a chance to show them how amazing reflexology can be. Of course, most people walking down the street have shoes on, so in my zealousness to practice, I began working on the hands of almost every new acquaintance.

Sharing my excitement with my younger sister one evening, I explained reflexology to her as I worked on her hands. She was impressed with how good it made her feel. Later, at a large, formal dinner party with my parents and some of their business associates, my sister and her new boyfriend were sitting across the table from me. In my overwhelming enthusiasm for my new skill, I blurted out to my sister, "Hey Brandi, have you given Tim a hand job yet?" At first I didn't understand the silence that came over the table. I've never used that term for a hand reflexology session again.

# In the Zone

To help illustrate how every part of our body is interconnected, we can compare our body to the globe we live on. The earth is one whole organism, just as our body is one whole organism. We affect the atmosphere by what we do on Earth just as we can affect our mind by having our feet worked on. However, just as the earth requires a map to help us define where we're going, you need a map of the reflex points of the feet and hands to understand and stimulate the areas you want to work on. Let's take a look at a couple ways to find our bearings.

There are many ways to chart or map the feet and the whole body. Charting or dividing the body conceptually into sections helps us understand how each section works. After we figure out all the sections, the whole makes more sense. On top of just mapping out the reflex points to corresponding organs on the soles of the feet and palms of the hands (see the figures earlier in this chapter), reflexology encompasses another theory: the belief that invisible pathways of energy run vertically along the body. These energy flows or lines are called *zones*.

To picture these zones, imagine your body tattooed with pin-stripes that run the length of your body from your toes on up to the top of your head, as illustrated in the following figure. These pinstripes are your zones. Working with these lines, and with points along the lines, is known as *zone therapy*.

**def•i•ni•tion**

**Zones** are invisible lines of energy that run longitudinally along the body. Working with these lines or sections is known as **zone therapy,** which many say is just another name for reflexology.

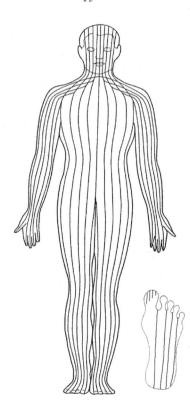

*Zone therapy divides the body into sections longitudinally. These lines of energy run through the body, affecting each organ along their path.*

It's important to understand the theory of zone therapy, because disease tends to run along these zone lines. For example, diabetes is a disease primarily caused by the malfunctioning of the pancreas. Take a look at the zone therapy diagram. The area where the pancreas lies is located between zones 3 and 4. Associated complications with diabetes include problems with the kidneys, which are also located along zones 3 and 4 (on both sides), and the eyes, which are also in zones 3 and 4.

Each zone or section acts as a kind of link to each organ or body part along the same meridian. A break or stagnation anywhere along these lines can disrupt the flow of energy to an organ, which may cause the organ to malfunction. Breaking up these blocked energies with applied reflexology sessions or zone therapy sessions restores proper energy and blood flow. This, in turn, helps restore proper energy to the organs.

## The Toe Bone's Connected to ... *What?*

Take another look at the zone therapy model. You can see how the outside of your feet represent the outer edges of your body, such as your thighs, hips, shoulders, and each side of your head. Conversely, the insides of your feet represent the middle zones of your body, such as the bladder, spine, and digestive organs on up to your nose.

Another way to see the body mapped out on the feet is to superimpose the entire body over the sole of the foot. In the following figure, you can see how the feet are associated with the parts of the body, from the head down to the lower bowel. The spinal column reflex area actually runs along the instep, so for some mental gymnastics, try to imagine this figure superimposed sideways, too.

*Here's an easy way to visualize the general reflex areas on the foot.*

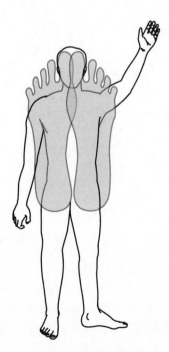

Now that you've learned about zones and reflex points, you can get a general idea of how affecting energy in one place can influence another. Just think of those zones as the overall map of electricity running up and down the body on a consistent basis. (I get into the actual foot and hand maps that correspond to specific organs and how you can use them in later chapters.)

# Ooh, That Tickles!

Many people think that letting someone touch their feet will tickle. Actually, when done properly, reflexology is anything but ticklish. To be effective, reflexology should be a fairly firm, deep pressure applied to the feet and hands. The pressure is administered slowly to avoid discomfort. The deeper you go, the slower you must apply pressure. Steady, flowing techniques are used. If anything, people feel tenderness rather than ticklishness in the feet with reflexology. The tenderness can feel somewhat like pressing on a bruised area.

## Where Does It Hurt?

Reflexology works by applying pressure to certain parts of the feet and hands, which stimulates the corresponding organs. The "tender" areas usually correspond to the organs that are sluggish. The tender spots on the feet and hands are the areas that actually need the most work.

Reflexology points may be tender because at any given time we have a certain amount of toxins flowing throughout our bodies. These toxins include cellular waste products, uric acid, pesticide residues, and other chemicals that the body cannot or has not eliminated.

### Tread Lightly

Toxins such as lead, mercury, aluminum, fluoride, chlorine, bacteria, and viruses have all been found in tap water. Avoid intake of these excess nasties by drinking only filtered water. Reverse osmosis water, in my opinion, is the cleanest, tastiest, and healthiest water for drinking, but a carbon filter is still a helpful way to filter some unwanted elements from tap water.

Toxic residues can linger inside us, sometimes indefinitely. Frequently, these toxins can settle along certain zones and cause interference with the energy flow to the rest of the organs along the zone pathways.

## Eliminating the Crunchies

Because most of us are either on our feet or have our feet lower than our heads most of the time, it is easy to imagine that, due to gravity, some heavier waste materials in our body settle at the end of our nerve endings on the bottoms of our feet. These areas are often referred to as deposits or what many refer to as "crunchies."

It has always been suspected that these crunchies consist of uric acid crystals, which is why, sometimes when you apply pressure to them to break them up, you can actually hear them crunch! It was thought that after these crystals are broken up, they can be carried off by the bloodstream and eliminated through natural elimination channels.

To finally get to the bottom of this conjecture, Dr. Jesus Manranares of Spain biopsied both crunchies and noncrunchy or regular reflexes on the soles of volunteers' feet. He found that, compared with the normal reflexes (no crunchies), *significantly* more nerve fibers and about half the connective tissue were found in the crunchy areas. About the same amount of blood vessels were in both.

So crunchies, when you find them, are mostly made up of nerve fibers, not uric acid. The inference to me here, too, is that when the body needs stimulation to a certain organ, the body learns to send nerve fibers to "congest" the particular corresponding reflex, crowding out the connective tissue to create a tender or tight area in the foot with the hopes that you'll find a reflexologist or at least go barefoot outside soon! This is also why when a reflex is worked, the hard texture breaks up and becomes soft while the tenderness subsides; signaling that the energy or signal (via the nerve fibers) has been sent along the meridian line to the corresponding organ to do its healing. Neat, huh?

Dr. Manranares is adamant that to continue to work on the reflex after this release is redundant. I agree, but that is why reflexologists can learn extra relaxing type techniques to soothe the client for an entire scheduled session even if all their crunchies have been broken up in the first half of the session.

You may experience a burning or even a poking sensation when these crunchies are breaking up. The discomfort should subside almost as fast as it came, though. Breaking up these congested areas and allowing the body to disperse them helps to restore proper energy flow to the zones and helps removes excess waste from the body, leaving you feeling refreshed and more vibrant.

# The Cure Is Underfoot

Reflexology is becoming a popular *holistic* therapy, at least in part because we're realizing that stress-reduction skills, good relationships, exercise, organic whole foods and clean water, fresh air, sunshine, herbs, and bodywork are all part of a fine recipe for robust health and preventative maintenance.

Reflexology goes hand in hand—or foot in foot—as the case may be, with other natural and medical therapies, which makes it that much more valuable. The therapies reflexology complements include the following:

♦ A solid nutritional and supplemental program

♦ Emotional/psychological counseling

♦ Bodywork of all types, including physical therapy

♦ Chiropractic care

♦ Acupuncture

♦ Aromatherapy

♦ Colonic irrigations

♦ Ear coning

**def•i•ni•tion**

**Holistic** is a term used to describe a way of living, practicing, or thinking that takes into account all factors of life. In holistic health, a practitioner considers the physical, mental, emotional, and spiritual aspects of the person to help them back to balance.

All these therapies can work together to create a holistically healthful lifestyle for you.

Reflexology is a therapeutic practice. Observing and working the reflex points can also give some clues to your state of health. Reflexology used in this manner lets you analyze what your health issues may be and can reinforce other holistic health assessments.

> **Tread Lightly**
>
> Although reflexologists are holistically oriented, don't expect them to be your only natural health therapist. No one can be a specialist in everything. Usually your reflexologist networks with others in the natural health community and can refer you to other practitioners to help you with things such as nutrition, herbs, psychological counseling, physical therapy, etc.

# Focus on Your Feet

Our feet carry us through life. They walk us down life's path. They bring us our independence. Are you walking the right path? The shape and condition of our feet can reflect if we are on the right path or even if we're afraid of walking this life path. Our feet give us the foundation upon which our whole body and, philosophically, our whole life rests.

Our feet bring us back to Earth and into our waking world when we get out of bed each morning. In our dreams, many times we fly or float. Our feet aren't important in the dream world, but in waking life, they keep us in our bodies, so to speak. Have you ever heard the saying, "I was so happy I was 2 feet off the ground."?

We jump for joy when we hear things that make us happy. But it's important to come back down and take care of earthly matters to keep balance in our lives. Our feet give us independence. They help us walk out of bad situations, run away from threatening circumstances, march to the beat of a different drummer, or even tiptoe through the tulips!

Reflexology is a very grounding therapy. "One step at a time" is a helpful saying to those of us feeling overwhelmed with too many projects to do. So many of us now live our lives almost entirely in our heads, constantly thinking, planning, talking, and dreaming. We need time to reconnect to our roots, and one of the best ways to get grounded and become centered is to concentrate on our feet.

The next time you're on a beach, take a barefooted walk in the sand and stop along the way and pick up seashells with your toes. This exercises the muscles in the feet. Notice how it makes you feel to walk in the sand. Or walk barefoot through some cold, wet grass early in the morning. These are both forms of natural reflexology and are also good therapies for the soul!

## The Least You Need to Know

◆ Reflexology maps out the connections between points on the feet and hands and the rest of the body.

◆ Using reflexology on the feet and hands positively affects all other parts of the body.

◆ The feet can give us clues to arising health problems and give us a chance to take preventative measures.

◆ Reflexology is a safe, natural therapy that complements all other holistic therapies.

# Chapter 2

# Why Do I Want My Feet Rubbed?

## In This Chapter

- ◆ Discover how to balance the body with reflexology
- ◆ Get prepared for detoxifying
- ◆ Use reflexology as an anti-stress therapy
- ◆ Learn who can and can't use reflexology
- ◆ Find out how often reflexology should be used

Now that you know what reflexology is all about, I'd like to fill you in on what makes it so good. Reflexology stimulates the body to produce those feel-good chemicals known as *endorphins*, and so far, I have found it to be the best way to get my family members to do big favors for me! It also ranks right up there as one of the best romantic gifts you can give your partner, especially in a pinch. Pin this thought under your cap: "Of course I didn't forget our anniversary, darling. Now lay back and kick off your shoes …."

Whether you're practicing on yourself or on someone else, this chapter helps you learn about some general uses of reflexology, fills you in on what you can expect, and even gives you inside tips about when and how often you can use this hands-on tool for health and happiness— and why you should!

# It's a Healing Feat

Reflexology is a natural way to stimulate healing in the body, and a healthy body is a body that feels good. Many folks are amazed at the instant relief they have from just a few minutes of deep pressure on the feet and/or hands. The hands are usually accessible, so you can work on yourself almost any time—in meetings, riding in a car (not if you're driving, please), watching a movie, getting your teeth cleaned—or virtually anywhere you have both hands free.

The ears also have reflex points, and most of us have our ears accessible all the time. The point is that reflexology can be used almost anywhere and anytime to promote balance and give you an instant lift or quick pain relief.

A reflexologist friend of mine was on a plane recently and was fortunate enough to be sitting next to a charming young lady about 7 years old. As the plane was descending, the girl began to experience excruciating pain in her ears because of sinus congestion. Instead of complaining about the little girl's cries, my friend, being the patient, healing woman she is, asked her mother for permission to work on her. The mother agreed, and my friend began to work on the girl's palms. Within minutes, the girl was drying her tears and feeling no more pain.

Now, if you're not lucky enough to be sitting next to a loving reflexologist the next time your sinuses are giving you grief, have no fear! By the time you finish reading this book, you'll be able to work on yourself for relief. In the meantime, check with your travel agent for specific seating arrangements or turn to Chapter 12 for more details about sinus reflex points on the hands and feet.

# Homeostasis: Getting It Right

My nutritional and holistic teachers over the years have all taught me the law of balance. It's only when we are imbalanced in some way, whether physically, mentally, or spiritually, that we experience ill health. I primarily address physical imbalances in this book, but keep the other two in mind for complete health.

Reflexology is great because it helps the body get and stay balanced. I'm not talking balanced as in walking on a balance beam. I'm talking about balance as it relates to the glandular functioning of your body, or *homeostasis*. Homeostasis is really a biochemical balancing act our endocrine glands play every day of our lives. Some of the functions controlled by homeostatic mechanisms are as follows:

◆ Heartbeat

◆ Blood production

◆ Blood pressure

◆ Body temperature

◆ Mineral balance

◆ Respiratory rate

◆ Glandular secretion

**def•i•ni•tion** _____

Homeostasis is the medical term used for the body's internal balancing act. It means that our unconscious body functions, such as body temperature and glandular secretions, are working for us to keep us alive and functioning.

Our glands all work together just like a smooth-running corporation. When one of the glands isn't up to par, the whole corporation suffers. This usually means extra work for the other glands as they try to make up the work left over by the slacker.

By using the reflex points on the soles of the feet and palms of the hands, we can send messages that can stimulate those glands that aren't keeping up and help the body become balanced again. For instance, symptoms of a sluggish thyroid gland could include unexplainable weight gain, lethargy, dry skin, and erratic sleeping patterns. These symptoms are signs that the body is out of balance.

More than likely, when your thyroid is out of balance and you rub your thyroid reflex point on the bottom of your foot, it will yell back at you—"*Ouch!*" Keep on rubbing—that's just the thyroid telling you it doesn't like getting caught sleeping on the job! (I explain how you can tell which areas or glands are sluggish in later chapters.)

It's not just the glands that can cause imbalance in the body functions. The major organs can become overloaded, tired, or injured; the muscles, skin, bones, hair, fingernails, joints, and all other parts of the body may show signs of imbalance. Bringing balance back to the body through stimulation is one goal of the reflexologist.

# Detoxing That'll Knock Your Socks Off

Most imbalances occur because of malnourishment, overuse or abuse, or too many toxins in the body causing irritations and sluggishness in certain areas. Detoxifying the body means doing some internal housecleaning. Believe it or not, our internal bodies get dusty and dirty and need to be cleansed periodically, just as our homes need a good spring cleaning.

The body has four main eliminative channels that serve as exit routes for waste products:

◆ The bowel

◆ The urinary system (kidneys and bladder)

◆ The respiratory system (lungs and sinuses)

◆ The skin

When the body or a particular organ is sluggish because of waste build-up, and then we stimulate that organ to get it back to work, it probably eliminates some toxins right away. This is called *detoxification*. When a body system is stimulated and gets stronger, it has the energy and ability to kick out toxins settling in it. You will know when your body is detoxifying because of the symptoms you experience.

Usually a full reflexology treatment stimulates all the organs and, therefore, stirs up a bunch of waste materials in the body. This is good, but you need to know what to expect when this happens to you!

## The Process of Elimination

One of the most common symptoms of the body detoxifying is a loosening of the bowels. Many necessary, quick trips to the bathroom will prove to you that you needed cleansing. This form of detoxifying after a reflexology treatment usually lasts no longer than a day. It's also a positive sign. You shouldn't try to stop this cleansing process by taking any medications that would cause constipation—let the cleansing begin!

---

**Tread Lightly** _____

Although cleansing of the bowel is a good sign, you shouldn't experience diarrhea after a reflexology treatment. A temporary cleansing due to a loosening of the bowel differs from diarrhea. Diarrhea can be caused by a viral, parasitic, or bacterial infestation that can dehydrate the body over a fairly short period of time and needs to be addressed.

---

The urinary system carries out waste products in the form of urine. The urine may be stronger smelling after a reflexology session, and you may have to visit the bathroom more often for a day or so after. This should also be encouraged. Drink plenty of pure water to help flush out the toxins.

## Sweating It Out

Sometimes when I work on someone with lung congestion, they experience a cleansing through the lungs, usually in the form of a phlegmy cough. I believe the reflexology treatment stimulated the lung's ability to loosen up old, hardened mucus, allowing for expectoration. So if you have copious amounts of mucus coming from your sinus passages or your lungs in the form of a cough after reflexology, you can count on this being a cleansing process.

Don't thwart the process by taking cough medications to inhibit your lungs from expelling the mucus. This only stops the cleansing process, which the reflexology treatment was designed to do in the first place! Instead, drink lots of water to speed up the process.

Foul breath is another strange symptom that may be experienced after a deep reflexology treatment. Again, this is due to toxins in the system, usually from the lungs, that have broken free and are leaving the body.

Detoxifying through the pores of the skin can show up as any type of skin eruption, including pimples, boils, rashes, or cold sores. Sweating during a deep treatment is sometimes experienced. This is the natural way your body rids itself of waste through the skin. When a treatment is effective in detoxifying, you shouldn't be surprised if your body odor changes for a day. In fact, after my first treatment, I smelled like maple syrup! Before I could panic about being nicknamed Aunt Jemima, the smell subsided.

# Stressed Out?

Reflexology promotes the body's production of *endorphins*—the feel-good hormones made by the pituitary gland in the brain. The flow of endorphins in the body acts on the nervous system to help reduce pain. Their effects on the body are similar to the effects of morphine.

I believe many of the painful symptoms we experience in the body are increased by stress. Stress tends to make us uptight. Literally, our muscles get tighter when we're under stress. Just think of yourself after having a confrontational meeting at work. Are your shoulders in your ears? Are your fists clenched? How about your jaw? Are you grinding your teeth or clenching them tight? These are all reactions to stressful situations, whether the stress is good or bad.

**def•i•ni•tion**

**Endorphins** are substances released by the pituitary gland that affect the central nervous system by reducing pain. Their effect on the body is similar to the effects of using pain-killing medications, such as morphine.

## Good Stress, Bad Stress, Ugly Stress

Some examples of "good" stress may be moving to a new, nicer home; starting a better job; getting married; or traveling to a new and exciting place. And of course we all experience the bad stressors, too, such as accidents, conflicts with others, financial worries, and so on. When the body and mind are adjusting to anything new, the muscles tighten in response, preparing for unexpected or new challenges.

But when we're stressed all the time, the effects can eventually tire us out. By using reflexology, we can help stimulate endorphins to relax the body, rejuvenate, and better tolerate the stresses of life. By utilizing reflexology as a stress-relieving technique, the body has a chance to relax the tight muscles that can cause pain.

> ### Foot Note
>
> There's something very deeply relaxing about a foot reflexology treatment. Most of the people I give reflexology to cannot stay conscious after a few minutes into their treatment and doze off or enter a trancelike state of relaxation. Many businessmen and -women I have worked on say they use their treatments with me as midafternoon catnaps that help them return to work feeling more creative and productive.

## A Balancing Act: Reducing PMS

Another form of stress is the ever-unpopular premenstrual syndrome (PMS). Fortunately, the stress, or tension, in the body can be released through reflexology. Reflexology has many effects on the body and can help balance the glands, reduce water retention, promote relaxation, and relieve pain by promoting endorphin production—all of which are important factors in relieving PMS symptoms.

The crankiness we feel when we're suffering from PMS is typically because the estrogen and progesterone ratio is out of balance, insulin sensitivity rises, the liver may be sluggish and having trouble processing out excess hormones, and the thyroid and adrenals also may be stressed, inhibiting their ability to help keep hormonal balance—i.e., being relaxed, happy, and content, and feeling like your normal self! Therefore, normal highs and lows that everyone goes through throughout the day affected by blood sugar levels, amount of sleep, stress, diet, exercise,

> ### Foot Note
>
> PMS symptoms are one of the most studied uses of reflexology. A Danish study in 1993 showed that reflexology proved to shorten the average duration of both PMS and menstruation.

etc. are intensified by these changing processes. By stimulating the glands to balance through reflexology, we can help make the highs and lows less drastic and help bring more harmony to the body.

Many times women hold excess water (known as *edema*) and feel bloated or puffy during certain times of the month. By utilizing the reflexology points on the feet, hands, and even ears, we can encourage the urinary system to cleanse, which can help release excess water. The effects are not only felt in the body as the swelling is reduced, but also have an impact on our emotional tension.

Obviously, reflexology has many uses for those of us suffering from any ailments or conditions caused by stress, tension, brain chemistry, or glandular imbalances. Relief of PMS is only one use, but it's one a large percentage of the population can appreciate. (I go into more detail in Chapter 15.)

# Gentle Enough for a Baby; Strong Enough for a Man

Reflexology is safe and effective and only helps the body do what it was designed to do anyway. So unless you're grossly negligent (or using instruments improperly), you really can't hurt anyone with reflexology.

If you're working on yourself, you know what hurts and what doesn't. When working on another person, you have to utilize your people skills to stay in communication with your receiver so you can push deep enough to get the desired results, yet still be gentle enough that they don't become tense. Later I cover the specific techniques and discuss how deep to go and so on, but for now, I want to talk about who can, can't, should, or shouldn't get a reflexology treatment.

> **Foot Note**
>
> Find a reflexologist and get a treatment for yourself so you can feel firsthand what reflexology is supposed to feel like. Then you can transfer that same feel into working on yourself between treatments.

Reflexology is one area in life where you should consider yourself first. Working on yourself is the best way to feel the effects of reflexology. For instance, I began utilizing this therapy as a crisis-management plan.

When something would hurt in my body, I would go to the corresponding reflex point, and sure enough, the reflex point would be sore. I would rub the spot every chance I got. As the pain went away in my body, the tenderness went away in my reflex point. Using the techniques on yourself helps you get in touch with your body and its functions.

## Kid Stuff—Working on Baby

Babies are especially responsive to reflexology. Many mothers instinctively rub their children's feet and hands when their children are cranky, crying, or uncomfortable. Reflexology works very well for little ones, as most babies enjoy being touched. Babies' feet have undeveloped arches, and their skin and bones are usually fairly soft. So don't dig too deeply into a baby's feet or hands! Gentle fingertip pressure is usually enough. Short, gentle sessions are most beneficial for infants: 10 minutes is usually sufficient. It's important not to overdo it when working with little ones.

Many times, gas pains, nausea, and general lethargy can be relieved when you rub a baby's feet or hands for several minutes. All the babies I have ever used reflexology on have fallen asleep after a few minutes of me working on them! This can be used as a trick for tired moms who need a break.

Babies also respond rather quickly to the detoxifying effects of reflexology. Therefore, this safe therapy can be used to help with gas pains due to constipation. I've found that the smaller the body, the faster the therapy works! So be aware that a child's reaction to most natural treatments can be almost instantaneous.

**Tread Lightly**

Baby's feet should not be worked on too deeply. A gentle but firm pressure while rubbing your baby's little feet and hands is sufficient. Results for babies are usually experienced immediately and can soothe a cranky baby or help relieve gas pains or constipation. Because the results can show up in a diaper, pack a few extra in the diaper bag!

# Who Shouldn't Use Reflexology?

Men and women of any age like the feel of reflexology and can use it without problems. However, pay attention to the person's pain tolerance. Someone who's generally healthy may not be very sensitive. If they already take good care of themselves and are used to other forms of bodywork such as massage, they may want or need deeper work to feel any real benefits.

**def•i•ni•tion**

A **contraindication** is a factor that prohibits a certain treatment for a specific patient due to some condition the patient has. Although reflexology is a safe treatment for almost anyone, it does have contraindications.

Every therapy has its own set of *contraindications*, and reflexology is no exception. Sometimes a therapy isn't recommended for someone with specific problems. I go over a more detailed list in Chapter 6, but for now, here are some general things to keep in mind when using reflexology:

♦ People with degenerative conditions such as diabetes or urinary system problems and the elderly can be very tender to the touch. Do not overwork these people.

♦ When working on babies, it's important to not overwork them. Use a very gentle pressure, and work no longer than 10 to 15 minutes for the entire treatment.

♦ Do not work directly on any injuries or foot conditions, and do not work an area that is painful to the touch.

♦ Do not overwork pregnant women, especially if they're prone to miscarriages.

# Reflexology and Pregnancy

The one serious contraindication for reflexology I always keep in mind is to work lightly on someone who is pregnant and who has had trouble carrying a pregnancy to term in the past. This could indicate that she lacks muscle tone in the uterus, and I would not want to stimulate a cleansing or stir up the circulation process. To be safe, I won't work on anyone who has had this problem before.

But don't let me scare off you moms-to-be! Typically, reflexology during pregnancy is a great way to gently relax the muscles and alleviate some of the tenderness in the feet that often comes with pregnancy. Many midwives offer reflexology treatments to help their clients through labor pains.

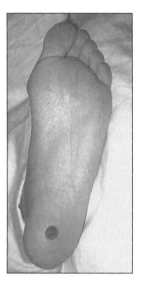

*This reflex is known casually as the delivery spot. It's actually a uterus reflex. When in labor, women can request that their partner deeply press and hold this spot for them on one or both feet. Midwives who are also reflexologists have shared that they believe this technique helps ease delivery.*

So for the future moms out there, here are my recommendations:

◆ Do offer gentle reflexology treatments to yourself or to your pregnant friends.

◆ Don't overstimulate the reproductive organ reflex points, unless you are working with someone in labor.

◆ Don't use reflexology at all on someone who has had miscarriages in the past or on anyone who is worried about miscarrying.

Although I do believe that reflexology is a wonderful therapy for pregnant ladies, the female organ reflex points should not be worked on too much. Neither should the foot be worked on too vigorously. We don't want to overstimulate the body when the body is busy building a new person!

# All Things in Time

The beauty of reflexology is that it can be used almost any time, as often as you wish, or as little as you want. Reflex points can be found on the ears, hands, and feet, so there's a good chance that at least one or two of these parts will be accessible almost all the time. Reflexology can be used as a quick pick-me-up or to facilitate instantaneous relief, but it's best used as regular therapy to promote overall balance and health.

I have found that, on occasion, the first reflexology treatment is not as effective as subsequent treatments. Sometimes this is because the receiver needs to get to know you a little better before they can relax totally and benefit from the stress-relieving effects of reflexology. Healing through relaxation is a big part of reflexology's magic.

For some, the first time you try reflexology you may just be breaking up some surface congestion, so you won't really notice any difference. If this happens to you, I suggest you try it again within a week. You may be surprised at what happens. Some of my best clients didn't have anything to say after their first treatments, but when they came back for a second time, they did experience results—and then continued to come back again and again.

Every body is different, and each person responds to reflexology in a different way. Sometimes the effect is more emotional than physical, although we should understand that all our emotions are actually hormonal/chemical reactions—which means there's little separation between emotional and physical, as every emotion either evokes or is evoked by physical changes—on a chemical level at least. But don't be surprised if you have someone burst into tears minutes after working on them. Reflexology can also be a cleansing process, and tears are one of the body's ways of releasing hormones, which aids in healing grief.

---

**Foot Note**

If you walk barefoot each day, you're giving yourself some reflexology stimulation, which is what we're naturally born to do. However, if you're getting reflexology treatments from someone else, you should always allow 24 hours between each reflexology session to give your body time to eliminate toxins released by the previous session.

## Use It Till You Lose It

How often should you use reflexology? The problem you're using reflexology to deal with will give you a clue. Although the therapy can be used as a stress reliever any time, some folks use it more seriously as a part of their regular health-care program. If you're working on a specific ailment or chronic problem, for instance, regular treatments until healing begins are the best way to start out. I always suggest, for chronic cases, that a person use reflexology once a week for 3 or 4 weeks or until they are feeling better, then maintain with bimonthly or monthly treatments. It's important to get the body balanced with several treatments up front and then maintain that balance.

## Speeding Up the Healing Process

Other natural therapies used along with reflexology can complement and dramatically speed the healing process. Consider coupling your reflexology treatments with any of the following:

- Colonic irrigations
- Herbs
- Vitamin, mineral, and enzyme therapies
- Proper nutrition
- Energy work
- Aromatherapy
- Counseling
- Exercise

All can make a big difference in getting healthy and then maintaining your health. Just like other natural healing therapies, using reflexology to bring your body back to health is effective, but it can take some time.

By the time you're not feeling your best, a lot of healing needs to take place before you can fully recover. Dr. Jack Ritchason, a well-known herbalist and nutritionist, says it takes five to seven times the normal amount of nutrition to build and repair as it does to maintain health. I believe this holds true for using all natural therapies. One reflexology treatment won't solve all your problems, just like one magic herb pill won't. Consistency is the key to getting where you want to be.

All in all, reflexology is an excellent, safe, efficient therapy that can be used on almost anyone, anytime, anywhere. Being so simple and safe, it can be integrated into anyone's lifestyle and serve as either a healing therapy or a preventative maintenance tool for health. It can even detect imbalances before you experience symptoms. Reflexology can help the body heal itself by detoxifying, de-stressing, and promoting homeostasis. To top it all off, reflexology can make you feel good, too.

These are all good reasons to get your feet rubbed. But before I address the techniques, let's dig up a little basics of foot anatomy in the next chapter.

## The Least You Need to Know

◆ Reflexology assists the body in healing by balancing glands, relaxing muscles, promoting pain-killing hormone production, and detoxifying the body.

◆ Reflexology can be used by almost anyone at any age.

◆ You can use reflexology as a natural healing therapy and as a preventative maintenance tool for health.

◆ Never work too vigorously or too deeply on a pregnant woman, a baby, or someone in a weakened state. And don't work at all on a pregnant woman who has had trouble in the past with carrying to term.

◆ Be patient when healing naturally. Your most recent symptoms may be the last to disappear.

# Chapter 3

# The Foot at a Glance

## In This Chapter

- ◆ Gain insight into the function and anatomy of the foot
- ◆ Understand how the feet serve as sensory organs
- ◆ Learn how to affect health through the pores of your feet
- ◆ Discover how your emotional health may be invisibly linked to your feet

There's more to the foot than meets the eye. I don't think most of us appreciate how much our feet really do for us. We depend on our feet, and if they don't feel good, we tend to take notice! Do you know that some people use footbaths to cure colds? Do you know how many bones are in your feet? Did you know that your feet can absorb substances you apply to them? Becoming familiar with the foot is key if you want to heal yourself (and/or others) with reflexology. So kick back, and let's take a step-by-step course through the anatomy of your amazing feet.

# My, What Big Feet You Have

The feet are literally the foundation for the body. They help us balance and give us a base on which to rest. The feet and toes are essential elements in body movement. They bear and propel the weight of the body during walking and running and help maintain balance when we change our body position.

> **Tip Toe** _____
>
> To see how the feet and hands are wired to the brain, try this exercise I call the Magic Finger exercise. Sit in a chair, and lift your leg so your right foot is off the ground in front of you. Rotate your foot clockwise. Continue doing this. Now with your right hand, point your index finger at your right foot and spin your finger in a counterclockwise direction. Wait! Don't change your foot direction! Can you do this? If you can, you have very good left/right brain integration; if you can't, then you must have a magic finger!

A strong foundation for the feet means that all the bones, ligaments, and muscles are in alignment with each other and functioning as a team. You may not be aware that your whole structural system and spinal alignment relies on the correct alignment of your feet, but it does! When the spine is out of alignment, you might experience any of the following problems:

- Headaches
- Lower back pain
- Neck pain
- Hip pain
- Sciatica (a pain beginning deep in the buttock and radiating down the thigh)

# A Bone to Pick

Are you aware that the bones in the feet and hands account for about half the bones in the entire body? The feet contain 28 bones each (26 main bones and 2 tiny bones called sesamoids), and the hands contain 27 each.

The bones of the toes are referred to as *phalanges*. The longer bones you see when you look down at the top of your feet are called *metatarsals*. The toes are also referred to as the *distal* part of the foot. This is easy to remember if you think of the most distant part of your foot being the distal part.

**def•i•ni•tion**

The bones of the toes are referred to as **phalanges**. The longer bones at the top of your feet are called **metatarsals**. The toes are the **distal** part of the foot.

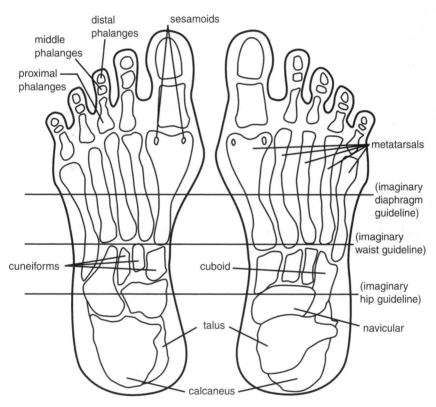

*The bones of the foot.*

## Tendon to the Muscles

Of course the foot is made up of more than just bones. Each foot has four muscle layers and about 33 muscles, which we give a real workout every day. While walking, it's estimated that the impact on the bottom of the foot equals about 900 pounds of pressure! Makes you really think twice about stepping on anyone's toes, doesn't it?

It's important that reflexologists learn about the 13 main tendons of each foot as well. Tendons are bandlike structures made up primarily of connective tissue that attach the muscles of the feet to the bones.

That bouncy spring in our step is facilitated by the arches that run lengthwise and crosswise over the foot. Some people have flat feet, which are caused by a lack of tone in the foot arches. (I discuss flat feet in more detail in Chapter 18.)

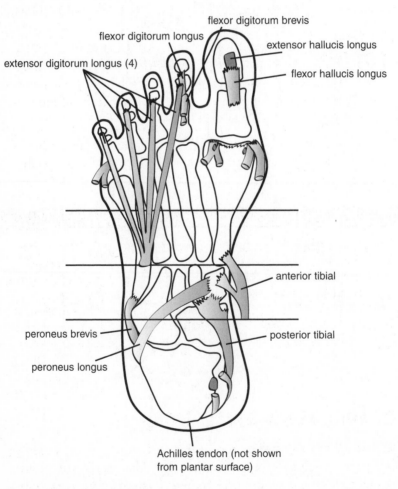

*The main tendons of the foot shown cut.*

## Foot Development

When we're babies, our arches are not developed yet, so we have flat feet. As babies begin to walk, the ligaments and muscles in their feet begin to form arches that help strengthen the bones in the middle of the foot. The arches in their feet are not fully developed until they are about 16 years old.

Not only does a baby's foot require walking for its correct formation and bone-building duties, but adults also need to walk to exercise and maintain foot bone strength and muscle tone. When asked if any exercises are particularly good for the feet, Glenn Copeland, D.P.M., simply states "Walking, walking, and more walking!" in his book *The Foot Book—Relief for Overused, Abused, and Ailing Feet* (Wiley, 1992). Proper care of your feet is very important—after all, your feet carry you everywhere you want to go. Many ailments of the feet—such as corns, calluses, and plantar warts—can all cause reflex problems to their corresponding body parts along the zones.

Take care of your feet by wearing proper shoes and getting adequate exercise such as walking, and your feet will carry you more steadily through life.

---

### Foot Note

One of the toughest clients I ever worked on was an ex-ballerina. She started dancing as a young girl, and her feet were literally deformed because of years taping her feet and wearing ballet shoes. She had her shoes bronzed as an heirloom, and it struck me how similar her feet were to being cast in bronze! The poor woman was always in pain. Obviously, our feet were not designed for this type of posture. But reflexology treatments helped the circulation in her feet and relieved a lot of her discomfort.

---

# The Foot as a Sensory Organ

The foot is a surprisingly sensitive organ that has the ability to sense subtle energy such as warmth, coolness, and other tactile sensations. The feet have thousands of nerve endings that send pulses of information from the feet to the brain (where all our motor skills are coordinated) and back again, all in split seconds.

Feeling and sensing through the feet is a natural occurrence we take part in every day. Have you ever noticed that if your feet are cold, the rest of your body feels cold? And how about when your feet are wrapped up inside a pair of hot, stifling boots on a sweltering day? What a relief it is when you can get those darn boots off and dip your feet into a crystal clear mountain stream. It really makes your whole body and soul feel good, doesn't it? You can see that we feel through our feet, and the feet affect how we feel.

**Tip Toe**

To see how the comfort of our feet changes our mental state, buy that someone who's always complaining of cold feet the plushest, softest, coziest pair of slippers you can find for a wintertime gift. Be there when they open them, and make them try on the slippers while you observe their facial expression. I bet they'll grin from ear to ear when they slip their feet into the slippers.

## Watch Where You Walk

The feet are really amazing. The soles of your feet contain some of the largest pores in the body, allowing your feet to absorb whatever is applied to them. Many reflexologists use pure essential oils before or after their reflexology treatments. When the oils are applied to the feet, they're absorbed almost immediately into the bloodstream and go directly into the cells, creating an oxygenating effect on the whole body. Many reflexologists are also aromatherapists and use oils that create certain therapeutic effects specifically for your needs.

**Tip Toe**

Do you apply lotions to your skin and feet? Because your skin has some absorbing properties, consider using lotions with natural ingredients such as fruits, vegetables, and herbal products.

Another great way to take advantage of the foot's efficient absorbing properties is by applying medicinal herbs or oils to the feet. One good use of this technique is by helping a child with a parasite infection. Unfortunately, parasites are not as uncommon as you may think. I recently read a statistic that claimed an estimated 95 percent of the world's population has some type of parasitic activity going on in their body!

Many moms have asked me how to rid their toddlers of these nasty pests. I always tell them that garlic has been used for hundreds of years to rid the body of parasites. You can crush a clove and apply it to the bottom of the toddler's foot. You can even keep the clove inside the bottom of their sock if it's not too uncomfortable for the child. As he walks on it all day, the foot absorbs the garlic's oil into the bloodstream. Daily application is recommended until the problem is gone.

## Footbaths—"Look, You're Soaking in It!"

For many years, natural health experts have been using therapies that treat the feet to change a body's condition. One I use frequently on my family and myself to help cure a cold or flu is a *footbath*.

### def•i•ni•tion

A **footbath** is simply the application of water, and sometimes essential oils, to the feet and lower legs to change the condition or circulation in the body. Because the feet are so sensitive to temperature, footbaths tend to work almost immediately and can be used before or after reflexology treatments, or any time you or a loved one is ill.

Specifically, footbaths work because of the temperature of the water. When we submerge our sensitive feet into a tub of cold water, the blood retracts from the lower extremities and retreats to the upper body. On the other hand, when we submerge our feet into a tub of hot water, the blood is drawn down into the lower extremities, away from the upper body. By understanding these actions, we can use footbaths to manipulate the circulation throughout the body and create certain therapeutic effects. The blood can act as a "flusher" of stagnant or congested toxins in the body or can promote healing to an area that's not getting enough blood.

If the head is congested, a cold footbath to stimulate the blood flow to the head area may help relieve sinus congestion. Using a hot footbath brings the blood to the feet and can relieve pressure-type pains, such as pressure headaches, in the upper part of the body.

# Foot Symbology: One Step at a Time

Do you have dreams with feet in them? The *symbology* of the foot infiltrates your subconscious mind and has meanings that are uncovered in your dream world. Check out Wilda B. Tanner's interpretation, from her fantastic book *The Mystical, Magical, Marvelous World of Dreams* (Sparrow Hawk Press, 1988), which I have used for years to interpret dreams:

> Feet represent foundation, belief, understanding, your ability to stand up for your rights or to put your foot down. May also imply taking the next step, stepping in the right direction, watching your step, one step at a time.

## def•i•ni•tion

Symbology or symbolism describes how a symbol can represent something else. Everyone has his or her own personalized set of symbolic meanings based on their life experiences. This is why you are the best interpreter of your own dream details.

If you're having any foot conditions or if you dream about foot conditions, think about the following list of foot symbolism and maybe take a holistic look at your problem. Of course you'll always want to rule out any medical conditions, structural, and/or endocrine imbalances first, but thinking in analogies can open your awareness about what might be going on subconsciously and help you master your thoughts and behaviors. The following list is compiled from my own teachings and integrates thoughts and symbols from Wilda Tanner's book and also Louise Hay's *Heal Your Body* (Hay House, 1994):

*Cold feet* symbolize a possible lack of courage to make the decision you know in your heart is right. Most of the time the *right* decisions are the hardest to make. Cold feet may imply you need to reconsider what you're getting yourself into.

*Flat feet* symbolize feeling a lack of support in your life. Or they can symbolize that you're afraid of not being able to support yourself or you're giving up your sense of self-reliance to take care of yourself. Flat feet can also mean that you feel a heavy responsibility in your life that you feel you can't support. It may also mean that you are a duck.

When you dare to go *barefoot*, you have the open understanding to be in touch with the earth, understand the basics of life, and are well grounded in your ideas and beliefs. Being barefoot means you feel a little vulnerable as well. If you can't bear to go bare, this may mean you feel you're unprepared for a situation or may symbolize that you can't tolerate or "can't stand" the situation you're in.

> **Tip Toe**
>
> It's fun to see how much a foot's shape can match the shape of the whole body. Some people have long, slender feet and toes and a long, slender body shape to match. Others are more curvaceous and have feet to match. Some folks with very wide big toes have a large head.

*Heel problems* may indicate that you're feeling susceptible to others' whims. Look closely at your relationships. Are you behaving like a heel?

The toes represent your mobility and balance as they relate to how you're walking through life. Toes symbolize the depth or extension of your understanding as they relate to the head area in reflexology. If you have *toe* problems, you might want to think about how you're proceeding on your path. Is your thinking clear? If you continue to stub your toe, is there something in your life you're not willing to face and really think about? Take a good look at what your mental focus is on. The toes can give you clues as to whether you're missing something or not.

Overall, the feet really symbolize the "earthy" part of us, the down-to-earth, physical side of our being. We stand from the ground up. Are your feet an extension of you, or are you an extension of your feet? In other words, might your foot problems be related to something else (nonphysical) that's going on in your life?

Recognizing this possibility is part of the solution; reflexology can help by easing any physical pain and by putting you in a more relaxed state of mind. In fact, reflexology sessions can sometimes lead to a release of pent-up emotions (something I discuss in Chapter 7), which, in turn, can be the beginning of an emotional healing process.

## The Least You Need to Know

- The feet and hands contain more than half the bones in the entire body.

- The foot is a sensory organ that can affect the feeling of the rest of the body and also absorbs nutrients.

- Footbaths can be used to get immediate relief from ailments such as head colds.

- The condition of the feet can reveal symbolic psychological factors that can help you take a look at your life situations and help you grow from them.

# 2

# Tools and Techniques for Feeling Good

Now that you understand how and why foot reflexology can be so good for you, you need to know how to turn a simple foot rub into a therapeutic reflexology session by implementing the proper techniques.

In Part 2, I walk you through the techniques so you can begin practicing your touch on the person who may have bought you this book—who most likely already volunteered with great anticipation to be your guinea pig! I also share with you some interesting ways you can look at the feet that might bring you a new appreciation for them, so get your fingers and thumbs loosened up and read on to get more in touch with yourself and your volunteers!

# Chapter 4

# Digging In: Where Do I Start?

## In This Chapter

- ◆ Prepare yourself to give your first reflexology treatment
- ◆ Learn to fine-tune your timing
- ◆ Discover the importance of a comfortable chair
- ◆ Get some tips on working the tender spots
- ◆ Learn a sample reflexology routine you can use

You've learned where most of the main reflexology points are and what the corresponding organs do for you, and now you want to prepare to get your hands on a partner, right? You've come to the right chapter. In this chapter, we take a look at how you get set to work on a mate, friend, or family member, and get a general idea of how a typical routine is performed. You need to know where and how to start, so let's take a look at the first steps.

# Taming Aunt Gretta

Whether it's speaking in public or practicing something new in front of others, we all occasionally experience a certain amount of stage fright. The same kind of freeze-up might occur the first time you practice reflexology on someone else. You might be especially nervous if you work on someone such as cynical, grouchy, old Aunt Gretta, who commonly refers to reflexology as "that witch-doctor stuff." (Note how she was willing to promptly whip off her beige-colored knee-highs, hop up on your chair or table, and let you practice on her anyway.)

Don't let her grouchiness intimidate you! After you're done with her, she'll be more soft and kind, and if you're lucky, she'll doze off and remember nothing while you get to practice. And at the worst, she'll have something more to complain about to the rest of your family, which is free publicity if nothing else.

This chapter gives you a basic orientation about how to give a reflexology treatment so you don't get caught staring open-mouthed and dumbfounded at a bare foot. The next two chapters help you learn the method to use for touching a foot and show you the typical "moves" and techniques to make your treatments effective and pleasant.

# Hand Me That Foot

Before we begin, I assume that after reading this book you won't go out and hang a sign on your door declaring that you're a reflexologist! This book is meant to be a natural and safe self-help book. It's also meant to give you some general tips for practicing on your friends and family. It can also be used as a reference guide, or even a prerequisite when you decide to take a hands-on course on the subject.

After reading this book and perhaps taking a bona fide course in reflexology, find some volunteers to practice on. At the next holiday gathering, stretch your fingers and seek out volunteers! Reflexology treatments make great gifts and can even help ease any family bickering that can spoil a good time. Your family and friends will be grateful, and you'll get some experience.

At home, you can have your partner lie in their bed or on a couch, or you can prop them up comfortably in a La-Z-Boy or other comfy chair. The important thing is that you're both comfortable.

Sit at your partner's feet, and for your best angle, their feet should be about central to your diaphragm. You will always want to use both hands when working on each foot. And keep your body centered around the foot you are working on. My normal treatments last about 1 hour, but you don't have to practice that long on someone to get results and make them feel good. Even 5 minutes with enough pressure on each hand or each foot makes a nice session and is a loving way to connect with a family member.

Remember that babies should not be overworked. A total of 10 minutes is adequate.

> **Tip Toe**
>
> If you're uncomfortable when giving reflexology to someone, you'll interrupt or distract from the session by constantly having to shift and fidget in an attempt to make yourself more comfortable. To avoid this, always situate yourself in a comfortable position before starting the session.

## Time for a Quickie?

Here's a quick 10-minute routine that covers both hands and feet and can be used on people of any age to get some quick relaxation and rejuvenation. With these moves, you won't be working any specific reflex points purposely, but you will be giving some general relaxation to the whole body. These moves are like squeezing the whole body and giving it a stretch—kind of like before you begin an exercise class.

Here's how to give a quick 10-minute reflexology routine:

After finding a place for your partner to lie back, be sure the back of their knees are supported with a pillow or cushion of some sort, so their back is not strained and their knees aren't hyperextended. (I emphasize this point over and over in this book.)

> **Foot Note**
>
> In Chapter 5, I describe the details of each technique, but to get you started, these few techniques are simple to understand. I've also referred to a few photos for further clarification.

Find yourself a comfortable chair or stool that positions you slightly lower than your partner's feet.

First, choose a foot and gently squeeze it with both hands, starting at the toes and working your way down to the heel (see Chapter 7 to get an idea of how to grasp the foot). Be sure you don't pull or pinch the skin while you're giving it this gentle squeeze. Repeat this move three times.

Rotate the foot on the ankle, using one hand to support the ankle while you hold the ball of the foot in the other hand (see Chapter 6). Rotate three times one direction and then three times the opposite direction.

Support the base of the toes by holding the ball of the foot, and with your other hand, grasp one toe at a time and gently rotate each toe three times in one direction and then three times in the other direction (see the "Tootsie Rolls and Rotating Toes" section in Chapter 6 for a detailed description on how to perform this move). Be sure not to pinch the toes too tight; you don't want to squeeze the toenail and make it uncomfortable. Grasp each toe tip just snug enough to hold on to it while you rotate it in a circular motion.

### Tip Toe

If you or the person you're working on has a headache, firmly squeeze the webbing between the thumb and first finger for up to 1 minute. This has often worked for my clients in less than 45 seconds. If the headache still isn't alleviated, try drinking a full glass of water.

Repeat these three moves on the opposite foot. This whole process should take about a total of 5 minutes to do both feet (2½ minutes each). The majority of the time is spent on rotating the toes.

You can spend another 5 minutes on the hands. Use your fingers and thumb to gently squeeze the webbing of one hand between the hand bones. The area between the base of the thumb and pointer finger feels especially good to most people (see Chapter 8 to locate the upper lymphatic reflexes). This area of the hand stimulates some of the upper lymphatics, the thyroid, the parathyroid, and even some of the bowel. Because this feels good to most people, you can spend a little extra time here.

Squeeze the webbing between the rest of the fingers one at a time. This works the upper lymphatics, chest/breast, and lungs. Finish off by squeezing each fingertip gently. This affects the brain and sinuses.

You should spend about 2½ minutes on each hand to complete a total 10-minute mini-treatment. At this point, your family member will probably beg you to take a reflexology class so they can be your practice volunteer!

## Timing Is Everything

Whether you're using this book to practice on yourself or family members, the timing of your sessions is important. The time you would like to spend working on yourself or others should be determined up front. This is easy for the professional, as they usually have a predetermined fee and time. However, when you're just experimenting with reflexology, you should determine the time you want to spend in advance and be sure you balance your work on both sides of the body. But you don't want to spend your time watching the clock.

There are different ways you can time yourself until you get comfortable with your own rhythm. You might want to consider using a kitchen timer. However, some people might be annoyed by the ticking sound of a timer, so if you use one, be sure the noise doesn't bother them. If it does, keep the timer outside the room you are working in so all you hear is the "ding" when you're done.

You can check the duration of a CD you choose to play during the treatment. Try to get CDs that match the length of time you want your typical treatment to last. You can coordinate a treatment to the length of the CD, which is a nice way to "conduct" business. This is especially true if the music has a type of crescendo in it. During the crescendo, you can do your most vigorous work and then drift back down into the relaxing techniques and finish up on the last note. It might sound corny, but if you give it a try, you might get into it!

> **Tread Lightly**
>
> Using any type of blaring alarm to signal the end of a reflexology treatment is not suggested. This will most likely annoy your partner and break them out of the euphoric mood you worked so hard to get them into.

You want to stay on track with timing so you don't spend too much time on one foot. If you run out of time, you won't be able to do an effective job on the opposite foot. This can leave a person feeling unbalanced. Reflexology relaxes the muscles in the body. You feel a difference in the side of the body that has been worked on. Therefore, to stay in balance, both sides should always be worked equally, whether you're working on yourself or a friend.

If you're working with only one point for a specific result, you should also work the same point on the opposite foot or hand. (Remember that most reflex points and areas are located on *both* hands and feet.) You can divide your treatment among the feet and hands any way you like. A good way to break down an hour treatment is to practice 20 minutes on each foot and then finish up with 10 minutes on each hand.

## Make Yourself Comfortable

When you and your partner have agreed upon how long the treatment will be, you must choose your location. Later I cover all the fluffy, atmospheric-type things that enhance treatments, but for now, I cover the basics of getting comfortable.

Whether your subject is sitting in a chair or lying on a couch, bed, or massage table, you want them to sit back and be comfortable or lie on their back. If the person is lying flat on her back, support her knees by putting a pillow under them and be sure her knees are slightly bent. Keeping the knees fully extended puts strain on the kneecaps and the back, which can cause discomfort. You don't want people leaving more uncomfortable than when they came in!

If you don't have a massage table or a reflexology chair to use, improvise by using a bed, a couch, or any type of chair your partner can recline in. Sit facing the soles of your partner's feet. After you ensure that your subject is comfortable, get situated yourself. Sit at the base of their feet and low enough that the tips of their toes are about level with your solar plexus. This position gives your body leverage if you're working on someone who requires deep work. (I talk more about specific finger techniques in later chapters.)

---

**Foot Note**

After a reflexology session, you can tell a difference in the receiver's body—and other people can see it, too! An experiment I use in classes to demonstrate this is to have my students work only on one foot as I explain the techniques: after about 15 minutes, I have them all stand and try to guess (on a different person) which foot was worked on. The hint is to look at the shoulders. Ninety-nine percent of the time, the shoulder on the reflexed-foot side of the body is significantly lower (i.e., more relaxed) than the opposite shoulder.

---

# Making Contact

One of the first things you want to do when working on someone is to establish contact with the foot. Gently lay your hand on one of their feet as you get yourself situated. Which foot you choose doesn't matter, but you'll want to touch the foot you intend to work on first.

You're making an initial contact to let the person know you're there. This first contact tends to put your subject at ease, especially if your touch is gentle, which it should be.

**Tread Lightly**

Be sure your hands are warmer than the foot you're working on. Eventually, both your hands and your partner's feet will warm up while you work, but you don't want them to jump at your first contact because of icy cold fingers! Try rubbing your hands vigorously together to warm them up first.

## Work Your Way Down

Now that you've got that foot in your hand, what do you do with it? One helpful hint is to start at the top of the foot and work your way down. This way you won't miss anything.

By the top, I mean the top to you, which from your vantage point will be the toes, known as the distal part of the foot. Work with each toe like it is its own separate little foot. The toes correspond to the sinus and head area. Many of us suffer from allergies. By working the toes first, you might just be able to give some immediate sinus relief.

Move on to the ball of the foot, down the body of the foot, and end at the heel. Then you can get the sides of the foot, and you won't forget anything!

The last part of this chapter outlines a longer routine for you to use. After you learn more specific techniques, you can refer to this outline as a general guide for giving a more in-depth session. By remembering to start at one end and work your way down, you'll cover all the territory.

## Come Down Off the Ceiling!

Everyone has his or her own level of pain tolerance. The levels different people can tolerate can be dramatic. One person may not even think you have started on them when you've been digging your deepest and exerting pressure into their reflex points, while another will practically jump off your table at the slightest amount of pressure!

> **Foot Note**
>
> Some people have high pain tolerance as a result of having experienced a lot of pain in their lives. They have developed a higher "pain threshold" to cope with the things they have been through.

Everyone is different, and you need to learn how to use enough pressure to be effective—but not brutal—to some sensitive tootsies. Likewise, you need to use your best judgment on how deep is too deep, even when your subject doesn't seem to be experiencing discomfort. Whether they tell you to go deeper or not, you should not go beyond what is reasonable pressure. If you have hands of steel, too much pressure could cause damage or bruising.

# Reaching the Depths of Your *Sole*

Just like in a relationship, you don't want to scare off someone by getting too deep too fast! Get to know your subject and their foot before you dive right into the depths of their soles.

Some other factors can help you decide whether to go deep or not and help you get a "feel" for your subject:

- Find out if the person has had reflexology before.
- If they have had reflexology before, ask what they liked about it.

- Find out if they especially disliked anything about their previous treatment.

- If they've never had reflexology before, ask them if they've had a massage.

- Question them on their preferences for deep or gentle massages.

The answers to these questions can help you determine how deep the treatment should be.

The condition of the foot can also give you a clue as to how deep you can go. For instance, if the foot is light in color, soft, and very flexible, you might not want to jump in deep right away. This person might have a delicate constitution and may not need or be able to tolerate a hefty treatment.

On the other hand (no pun intended), a foot that looks like it has been barefoot most of its life and is heavily callused may need deeper work to be effective. This is not always the case, however. Going slowly is your best bet, and be sure to ask your subject to tell you if the pressure is uncomfortable or if you need to go deeper.

### Tread Lightly

As with anything, looks can be deceiving. I have worked on feet that appeared to be delicate and sensitive that were just the opposite. On the other hand, a few very callused feet have been very sensitive to my touch! You never know, so be sure you customize your pressure for the receiver and not by your own preconception!

## Down to the Bone

Some areas of the foot are not appropriate to work deeply. You never want to work deeply directly on a bone or on the joints. When I talk about deep pressure, I generally mean working on the foot's muscle layers. The ball of the foot and the heel are sometimes callused and harder. Therefore, to be effective, you can probably apply more pressure to these areas. The mid-part of the foot contains the majority of organ reflex points and you can vary the pressure.

**Tip Toe**

Some people won't be comfortable taking off their socks. That's okay. You can work on your own or another person's feet through the socks. However, if the socks are dirty, offer them a clean pair to make the treatment more pleasant for you.

You don't want to go deep enough to give your subject a cramp! This may happen when you're working on the instep. If it does, help them stretch out the cramp and then go back to the instep more gently. The deeper you work, the *slower* you need to apply pressure. You don't want to make anyone feel like they just stepped on a rock. Applying the pressure slowly allows the body time to adjust.

## That Feels Yummy: A Relaxing Technique

Remember that pain causes tension, so anytime we have discomfort, we want to re-relax the body. Yummies, a reflexology technique so named by my first reflexology teacher, Isabelle Hutton, is a good way to do this.

Yummies is a technique whereby you place both of your palms on either side of the ball of the foot and gently but vigorously move your hands in opposite directions, rolling the foot loosely between your hands. In this technique, one hand goes forward, or away from you, while the other hand moves toward you. Repeat this motion for about 5 to 10 seconds, and be sure your hands don't slide on the skin to prevent friction "skin burn." This technique relaxes the body, especially the ankle and calf muscles.

*Yummies is a technique of rubbing the ball of the foot back and forth between both hands.*

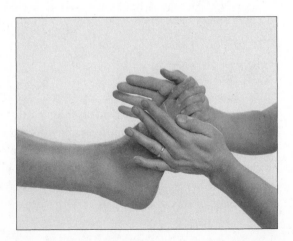

**Tread Lightly** _____

If you cause someone to yell when hitting a tender spot, don't allow your hands to jerk away from them, but follow this regimen: stop pushing, back off slightly, and hold the spot for a moment. Their body will adjust to the pressure. Then give them a yummy, which tends to make them forget they ever had any discomfort!

# When Your Feet Bruise

If your subject has a tendency toward anemia or if they bruise easily, work more gently on them. You don't want them to go home with bruises, even if the treatment felt good. I had a client tell me that her first reflexology experience with another practitioner was effective but brutal. After her first treatment, she could barely walk the next day, and she had bruises up and down her shins for 2 weeks! When I asked her why she wanted to get another reflexology treatment after that experience, she said she felt the treatment helped the rest of her body feel better anyway.

A full assessment on this woman showed her to have a low red blood cell count, and she also bruised very easily. Therefore, I didn't work on her vigorously, but I was effective enough to keep her coming back for more. We also worked with her nutritionally, and she began taking an algae supplement, liquid chlorophyll, and yellow dock to feed her body extra herbal sources of protein and iron, since anemia is associated with a lack of these nutrients.

The program changed her appearance and vastly improved her energy levels. The dark circles under her eyes went away, and she enjoyed her newfound energy. Eventually, I was able to work much deeper on her feet without any bruising.

**Tip Toe** _____

I find that my women clients are more sensitive to reflexology just before their periods and not as sensitive during other times of the month. I have to adjust my pressure to fit the need at the time. You will become aware of this for yourself, too.

Another good question to ask someone before you start working on them is if they have any old foot or hand injuries. Never work deeply on old injuries. I learned this lesson firsthand with someone who asked me to demonstrate reflexology on him at a luncheon. I acquiesced until his hand began to turn red and swell!

Embarrassed, I apologized and attempted a getaway. He then told me that he had injured the hand 20 years ago. His inflammation subsided, and he reported a renewed flexibility thereafter! Could it have been that my short use of reflexology was just what his hand needed to complete healing? No matter—please learn from what I did with this experience:

◆ Always ask about old injuries before starting.

◆ Never begin working haphazardly on someone.

◆ Never work too deeply on an old injury.

## Smoothing the Way

Occasionally you'll run into someone who, no matter how hard you push, no matter how deep you go, always asks you to go deeper. Many times these people have a lot of calluses built up on their feet. This makes it harder for you to work on them and also makes them less sensitive to your treatments.

Suggest that they purchase a pumice stone and use it to rid themselves of their built-up calluses. The pumice treatments help make the feet more supple and sensitive to treatments.

My aunt Alice, a nationally certified reflexologist, has another trick up her sleeve: she offers her clients a foot wax dip before their reflexology session. She says these hot wax treatments not only make the feet feel fantastic, but also serve to exfoliate the skin and soften it up before reflexology.

## The Tender Spots Need Work

As you begin to work with reflexology, you'll notice that you'll find tender areas on the feet and hands. Besides indicating any local problems (such as corns or warts), these tender spots generally are the areas that need the most work. When there's tenderness in an area, there's usually corresponding congestion in the organ associated with the reflex point.

Many times you'll be able to tell where the tender spots are because you'll be able to feel crunchies in those areas. Sometimes you'll feel "electrical sparks" shooting out of a particular point. When you feel these crunchies or sparks, you might want to ask your subject if they can feel any particular sensation.

---

### Tread Lightly

If part of your foot has an injury, infection, bruise, or other type ailment, do not work directly on that spot. The same holds true for any-one else you work on. You can, however, work around the injured spot, which still moves lymph and circulation and can enhance healing. You can also work on the corresponding hand instead of the foot if the foot is injured, or vice versa.

---

Occasionally a person will tell you that you're digging into them with your fingernail. Of course, you have trimmed your nails already (I cover the importance of keeping short nails in Chapter 5), so it won't be your nail they feel. They also might ask you what type of tool you're using when you hit one of these crunchies.

What they're probably feeling is the sensation of the nerve fiber bundles being broken up in their foot. It's not you at all, but a release of built-up energy congestion that has accumulated in the foot. You can work on these areas until the tenderness subsides. This sometimes can be done in one treatment, but it might take as many as three in a week to get rid of the pain and stimulate the corresponding organs into action.

In Part 4, where I go into more detail about tender spots and precautions, I talk about when tender spots are not appropriate to work on. If you want details of some of the contraindications (when you shouldn't use reflexology), see the table in Chapter 6, which lists all the warnings for reflexology. But for now, the tender spots are your clues that they need to be worked!

# A Typical Routine

Now that you're starting to get comfortable, let's walk through a typical reflexology treatment. This is the first routine I learned early in my career, with some of my own refinements added. You can use this to practice on friends and family who volunteer to let you work on them. After you learn all the techniques, you can come back to this treatment and use it as a guide.

You can use a typical routine like this for as long as you like, but because we're all creative beings and each person you work on will have different needs and requests, you can probably change this routine over time. I like to perform a generalized routine on each new person. When and if I find especially tender areas, I work on those areas until the tenderness subsides. Put your own creativity into your work, and soon you won't be worried about what to do next!

Begin establishing rapport with your subject, and make a gentle contact with the foot. Question them about any injuries to the feet or hands you need to be aware of. Make a general survey of the foot, ankle, and lower leg. Note any complaints the person has.

After grasping a foot with one hand, begin working on the big toe with the other hand. Always use a supporting hand to support the work you are doing with the other. This gives you more depth, effectiveness by focusing your pressure. The big toe corresponds to the head area, and some people will even feel goose bumps on their scalp as you work on the toe. Proceed to the small toes, which cover the brain, sinuses, eyes, and ears. Work your way to the ball of the foot, which corresponds to the lung and heart area.

### Foot Note

Research scientists have found actual energy "spots" or areas that are different from normal energy (kind of like concentrations of energy) located under the skin at certain acupressure and acupuncture spots along the body. Some of these may be found on the soles of the feet. Researchers are using the acupuncture areas versus reflexology areas to try to validate this energy's existence; however, some acupuncture and reflex areas overlap, so keep your ears open to hear more on this exciting subject. Isn't it fun when science catches up with ancient beliefs and validates them for the skeptics?

Work on the thyroid area, which is found all around the base of the big toe. Next, work your way down the spine reflex and along the instep of the foot. The hip area is next—work your way from one side of the foot to the other. Cover each of the gonad points on either side of the ankle, and work across the top of the ankle to connect both points.

Then go back to the middle of the foot, working all the digestive and intestinal organs. Finish up the feet by "milking" the legs from the knees down, and shake out the extra energy (see this technique in Chapter 5 in the "Shake a Leg" section). Proceed to the hands for a complete treatment.

Leave the recipient to rest, and go wash your hands. Come back with a glass of pure drinking water for your receiver, and ask them how they feel.

The next chapters give you the actual finger and hand techniques you will use in this routine. Soon you'll get really good at this.

## The Least You Need to Know

◆ Before you get started, decide what kind of treatment you'll perform (hands, feet, or both), how long it will take, and what position will be most comfortable.

◆ When you first start practicing reflexology, start at the top of the toes and work your way down. This ensures that you cover everything.

◆ Everyone has a different level of pain tolerance. It's up to you to use your common sense to determine how much pressure is enough.

◆ Always ask your subject if they have had injuries to the feet or hands before you begin working on them.

◆ Come back to the typical routine in this chapter when you have learned the actual finger techniques laid out in the next chapters, and use these techniques until you develop your own style.

# Chapter 5

# Let Your Fingers Do the Walking

## In This Chapter

- Learn some of reflexology's basic techniques
- Find out how to grip and support the foot
- Discover the joys of finger walking and thumb nibbling
- Understand how to read your partner's facial clues
- Practice some lower-leg moves to complement a treatment

Foot rub, foot job, foot massage—you know for sure that a qualified, professional reflexologist will *never* use these terms to describe their practice. Actually, there's very little rubbing or massaging in a reflexology session. So although it might rub you wrong when a potential recipient asks you for a foot massage, politely correct them on their semantics and then demonstrate how a *real* reflexology session is supposed to feel!

This chapter lets your fingers do the walkin' as we practice together some real reflexology techniques. After a bit of trying this on yourself, your positive attitude should be the only thing that rubs off!

# You're in Good Hands

Always use both hands in reflexology. Remember, your goal is to help the person relax completely. They can't do this if you're not supporting their feet or hands to stop them from moving away from your pressure. Gently support the foot from one side while you work with your finger and thumb techniques on the other.

For instance, if you're using a thumb-walking technique (I get to that in a minute) for the urinary system, which covers mostly the inside middle of the foot, thumb walk with one hand while you support the opposite side of the foot with the other hand.

*Grasp the opposite side of the foot while working the urinary system reflexes.*

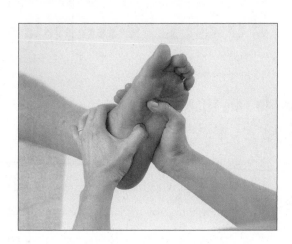

![Tread Lightly icon] **Tread Lightly** _____

If you have a hand or finger injury, don't perform reflexology on yourself or others until you heal. You cannot be effective with an injury, and you may injure yourself further by applying pressure to an injured hand. You might want to use some tools on yourself, such as a foot roller, until your hands/fingers recover fully.

Use your supporting hand to secure the foot as close as possible to the area you're working on. For example, if you're working on the lung area (on the ball of the foot) with a thumb technique, use your other hand to support the top half of the foot.

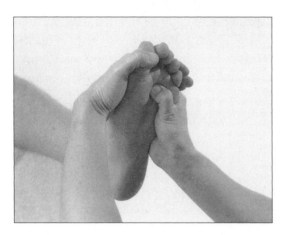

*Support the opposite side of the foot while working on the lung reflex area.*

Don't worry about not having big, strong hands or fingers for reflexology work. As you perform reflexology techniques, your hands will strengthen naturally.

**Tread Lightly**

Keep your fingernails and thumbnails very short so you can use your fingertips—not your fingernails—to stimulate reflex points. Sorry ladies, but long fingernails just don't work well with reflexology. Keep them trimmed, and be sure the edges are well rounded so you don't cause yourself or your subjects any discomfort.

# Finger Walking

Now let's take a look at some of the basic reflexology techniques. Reflexology is honest and straightforward, and so is its terminology. I like the simplicity of the reflexology terms, because they describe the technique and say exactly what they mean. The first one we'll look at is called *finger walking*, which is just what it sounds like.

The finger-walking technique is utilized in areas where it would be awkward to use the thumbs. Most of the techniques will feel very natural to you as you use them. For finger walking, you use your fingers, mostly your pointer finger.

To get in position, put your hand out in front of you (left or right hand, whichever you're most comfortable with). Place the pad of your middle finger on top of your pointer finger nail pad. You will have effectively made a shape that resembles a capital D.

> **Tread Lightly**
>
> When you perform this technique on yourself or others, don't drag your wrist across the foot. Keep your wrist level with the rest of your hand.

Apply the tip of your pointer finger on the area of the foot or hand you want to work, and use your middle finger to push down on the pointer finger to apply pressure. The walking begins as you inch your way across a reflex.

If you imagine that your hand is dead weight—meaning it's detached from your wrist and the rest of your arm (like "Thing" from the television show *The Addams Family*), you can exaggerate the finger-walking technique by pulling or inching your hand along a flat surface by just using these two fingers. The primary pressure is under your pointer fingertip.

One of the primary uses for this technique is to walk around the top part of the foot from ankle to ankle. This area represents the fallopian tubes in women or the spermatic cord in men (see Chapter 15) and also the pelvic area. If you were a massage therapist, working this area would correspond to massaging the lower back from one hip to the other.

This area is good to work when a person has a sore lower back, sore hips, menstrual cramps, or any type of reproductive problem. Start from the middle of one side of the heel (around where the ovary/testes or uterus/prostate points are) and "walk" the fingers forward over the top of the foot to the other side of the heel.

Another way of using finger walking to work this same area is to hold the foot with both hands and place each pointer finger in the finger-walking position on either side of each ankle (on the inner and outer ankle where the ovary/testes and uterus/prostate points are). In this position, your thumbs are under and below the heel of the foot. You can simultaneously finger walk up both sides and around the fallopian tube/spermatic cord reflex, with your fingers working their way toward each other. You'll end when your fingertips come close to meeting in the middle (at about the top of the ankle). Just be sure not to pinch the skin when your fingers meet at the top!

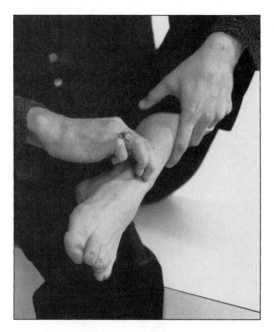

*Finger walking around the fallopian tube/pelvic region using a one-handed technique.*

Three main areas for using finger techniques are as follows:

♦ For the fallopian tube/lower pelvic region

♦ For toe/finger squeezing

♦ For squeezing or walking along the lymphatic reflexes

There are no strict rules about when to use the fingers versus the thumbs, and you can use both all over the feet, ankles, hands, wrists, and wherever is comfortable.

## Tip Toe

In reflexology, your hands are your tools. Take good care of them, and never do anything that's painful to you when performing reflexology.

If you have arthritis in your hands and cannot perform reflexology on yourself at home, consider utilizing reflexology rollers, machines, or other tools between getting sessions from a professional.

*Finger techniques for working the toes. This technique can also be used for the fingers in hand reflexology.*

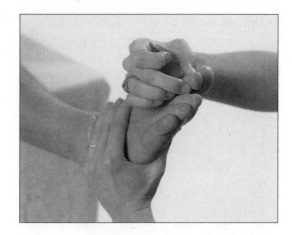

*Finger walking along the lymphatic system on the hand.*

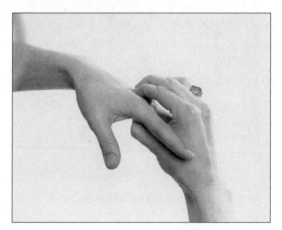

# Thumb Nibbling

*Thumb nibbling* is a term I use for the thumb technique that corresponds to finger walking (the correct term is *thumb walking*). Reflexologists use the term to describe a common technique that utilizes the thumb to stimulate reflex points.

The thumb is the most often utilized finger when giving treatments. The thumb is short and stout, which seems to give it more strength, and it can be used to stimulate those points that need deeper stimulation. Rolling the rest of your fingers into a loose fist and keeping your thumb close to your fist gives your thumb more strength and leverage for some of the stimulation points you use.

**Tip Toe**

A tennis ball–size rubber ball makes a great hand exerciser and stress reliever. Squeeze the ball for a few minutes in each hand daily to build hand strength and keep your joints flexible. Here's a tip for stress relief: buy some Silly Putty, roll it into a smooth ball, and press on a silly cartoon face or just poke a face into it. Then name it. Mine's name is Mr. Pulaski. When I squeeze Mr. Pulaski it cracks me up and eases stress.

Thumb nibbling sounds just like it works. The face of the nail always points forward when thumb nibbling. You can pretend that the top of your thumbnail is like PacMan eating his way across the crunchies of the foot!

Using the corner of your thumb to pinpoint deeper areas is good as long as your thumbnails are rounded. When you use the thumb or finger techniques, always "walk" with your fingernail in a forward motion (away from you). You'll find that this feels pretty natural.

Be sure, however, that you're *not* using your thumb joint for leverage and pressure. Instead, use your whole arm for leverage to dig the thumb into the reflex. When you nibble with your thumb, think of your thumb as a bottle opener. Place your thumb in position, bent at the joint. Then rotate your *wrist* back and forth to make the movement. In other words, you don't want your thumb moving at the joint like an inch worm, but instead, it should mostly stay bent while your wrist does the moving. (You can rest the fingers you aren't using on the opposite side of the foot when you're working in this location.)

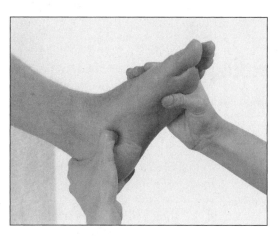

*Thumb walking along the spine reflex.*

You utilize thumb walking on the central nervous system reflexes, the digestive system reflexes, the intestinal system reflexes, the urinary system reflexes, and the respiratory areas.

# Pain Is Not Gain—Usually

Really, pain is not gain in anything we do—but a little discomfort sometimes helps us grow. Unless there's a local problem such as a corn or a wart, the tender spots on the reflex areas are the areas that need to be worked. In Chapter 4, I talked about the fact that everyone has his or her own pain tolerance levels, and you need to be sensitive to them. But to be effective, you need to stir up a little discomfort every once in a while!

The pressure you exert when giving someone a treatment should be firm but not painful. Tender, like the almost-pleasant pain of a muscle ache or minor bruise, is okay. Pressure should be administered as deeply as the person can tolerate to be most effective. Check out Chapter 4 for more pointers.

Some people react to discomfort by saying "Wow, that's tender!" but if they say "*Ouch!* That *hurts!*" you're going too deep. Or if you're a greenhorn, you might have inadvertently pinched the skin. You can also read the faces of the folks you're working on for a clue. This is especially true if you're using a chair and can see their faces when you work on them.

If the person you practiced reflexology on has a relaxed smile on his or her face when you're done, you probably did a good job. If you see that you're causing someone pain or discomfort, back off on how deeply you're working. Too much discomfort can bring out the worst in anyone!

# Hooked on Reflexology

The preceding section should have given you a pretty good sense of how deep you can go and how to tell when to ease up. Now we're going to look at a technique that requires you to go pretty deep—which usually gets a distinct response.

*Hook and back up* is a technique mostly performed on those tough-to-reach reflexes, such as the pituitary and pineal gland points (see Chapter 11). They are glands in the brain, and their reflex points are located in the middle of each large toe, in the head area. These glands regulate myriad functions and are a popular spot to work on. Being endocrine glands, these glands also have a great influence on our hormones.

To access these points, you need to "hook" your thumb into the location and then kind of pull upward and inward to stimulate the point, as shown in the following photo. This can be difficult to do, especially if you have fairly flat thumbs like I do. This is why some reflexologists use a tool with a pointy, but soft rubber tip like an eraser on the end of a pencil to find these points.

To learn to do this technique with your thumb, you just have to keep practicing until you get it. You'll know when you've found the pituitary and pineal spots because of the "electric shock" you'll feel if you're working on yourself. If you're working on someone else, no doubt your subject will tell you about it.

> **Tip Toe**
>
> The pineal and pituitary glands are endocrine glands that regulate a host of functions in the body and may be helpful in regulating weight and controlling water retention, insomnia, and hormonal imbalances associated with PMS: acne, bloating, moodiness, and cravings. They're also used for dream enhancement.

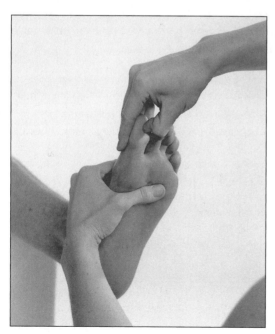

*The hook and back up technique. Use this technique to stimulate the pituitary and pineal reflexes. Be sure to support the toe firmly (not shown).*

# Milk It for All It's Worth

A common technique for ending reflexology sessions is called *milking the leg*. It can only be done if you're working on someone else; this one isn't a self-help technique, but it's nice for the person you're doing it to.

Milking the leg is done just after you're done giving a complete reflexology session on the feet. Starting just below the knee, wrap both hands around the calf. Gently squeeze both of your hands at the same time, loosen them a bit, slide your hands down the leg toward the foot a few inches (without removing your hands), and squeeze again. Continue this process all the way down to the ankle, foot, and toes. This should take you about 5 to 7 "squeezes," depending on how long the calf is.

You can work your way down, squeezing the foot in the same manner, and then "pull off" the energy at the tips of the toes with a grabbing motion. The best way to describe how to do this is to imagine that the person's leg is a rolled up, sopping wet towel. Your job is to squeeze the towel gently from the top all the way down, pushing all the water toward the end of the towel (the foot) and then pulling off all the excess water at the bottom.

This technique is meant to cleanse a person's energy field, in addition to being relaxing to the body. Use this method to help pull out all the negativity and stress from a person. Then, after you're done milking the leg, it's time for a milk and cookie break!

---

### Foot Note

Milking the leg is a technique designed by one of my reflexology teachers as an extra treat for her clients to cleanse negative energy and to revitalize the entire leg. As such, this technique may not be covered in any reflexology classes you take. Just as each reflexology chart you see will differ slightly, every teacher will have his or her own unique ways of teaching. So don't expect all classes to be completely identical, although most of the basics will be uniform, especially as the reflexology community begins to adapt specific standards. However, if you're lucky, you'll get to learn some specialty moves from your instructors after you learn the basics.

## You're Pulling My Leg

To stretch the lower back and help the person feel more relaxed after a reflexology treatment, you can gently pull on each leg. To do this, be sure to use both hands. When the person is lying flat on his or her back, simply grasp the underside of his knee with one of your hands and hold the bottom of his heel with your other hand. Gently use your own body to tug softly at your subject's leg. You can do this by leaning your body back slowly in your chair.

This technique makes the person feel that you have lengthened their leg a bit. Be sure you do the same to the opposite leg. Balance is important!

You can also shake the leg at this point, which is described in the following section.

## Shake a Leg

*Put your left foot in, take your left foot out, put your left foot in, and then you shake it all about! Do the hokey pokey and we turn ourselves about ... that's what it's all about!*

Not that I would consider reflexology hokey pokey, but shaking the leg at the end of a session sure seems to relax the entire body and is a nice way to end a treatment. This technique is done very gently, and you need to support the knee while you do it so you don't put extra *torque* on the knee. By torque, I mean any strain on the knee that makes it bend in a way it isn't designed to bend! This includes side to side and backward.

**def•i•ni•tion** _____

**Torque** is a turning or twisting force. In reflexology, you need to be careful not to torque the knee, because it's only designed to bend one way.

Support the back side of the knee with one hand, and rest the person's calf along the underside of your forearm. With your other hand, hold the bottom of the heel. With both hands, begin to gently shake the leg top to bottom and then side to side.

When you shake a leg side to side, you use the movement of your upper body more so than just your arms and hands. This helps keep the movement gentle and the range of movement smaller.

*The shake-a-leg technique. Be sure to support the knee when leg pulling or leg shaking. This technique is a great way to end a session.*

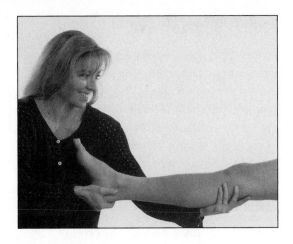

This is sure to be a hit with your subject. It helps relax the whole body and can even ease tension in the lower back and hips.

Now you've learned how to support and grip the foot, found out how to finger and thumb walk, learned a few moves, and saw some general relaxation techniques. Let's now build on all this knowledge in Chapter 6, where you can really polish your skills and learn plenty more moves. Let's go!

## The Least You Need to Know

- ◆ Reflexology's terminology matches the techniques and is quite straightforward and easy to remember.

- ◆ Always use two hands when performing reflexology. One hand must always be supporting the foot or hand you're working on.

- ◆ When using your thumb techniques, curl the rest of your fingers in. This lends the thumb more strength and support.

- ◆ Take clues from the person you're working on to determine how much pressure you should exert. Pressure should be as deep as can be tolerated.

- ◆ You can finish your treatment by gently pulling, shaking, and milking the legs from the knees down to enhance flexibility and relaxation and help clear negative energies.

# Chapter 6

# How to Touch

## In This Chapter

- ◆ Gain insight into the subtleties of touch
- ◆ Discover the importance of maintaining contact
- ◆ Learn some circular and rotating techniques
- ◆ Know what to do when working with an injured or ailing foot
- ◆ Learn the major contraindications for reflexology

Are you one of those people, like me, who love to have your feet rubbed? When I get a massage instead of reflexology, I ask the massage therapist to concentrate on my neck and then my feet. Even though she may not be a reflexologist, having my feet touched feels fantastic and relaxes me more than anything. However, after you've experienced a reflexology session from a trained and skilled reflexologist, you'll understand the powerful difference between reflexology and massage. You'll also understand the differences between a professionally trained reflexologist and your partner who occasionally rubs your feet as a loving gesture. (Not that you should pass up that opportunity!)

Massage works on the muscles and tendons and is a wonderful therapy, but reflexology works on energy, zones, and reflexes of only the feet, hands, and ears, and is a different experience. Let's take a closer look now at some of the similarities massage therapists and reflexologists *do* share and then we'll go into detail about when reflexology is *not* appropriate.

# A Healing Touch

Touch is a very important aspect of our lives, central to reflexology in the same way it's important to touch the ones we love. Although you can use reflexology on yourself and gain beneficial results, having an experienced reflexologist work on you is an unsurpassed experience. When you work on someone or have someone work on you, an energy exchange takes place between the therapist's hands and the recipient's feet.

---

### Foot Note

A teacher once encouraged my classmates and I to use our intuition when giving reflexology, keep our ego out of the way, and work the areas we "sensed" needed the most work. I find myself doing this with my clients at times. Something just tells me I need to work a particular spot. When I go to the spot, my client usually looks at me and asks, "What's that?!" in response to the change in the feel of the area I work. I can't verify it, but I assume these intuitive areas reflexologists learn to detect with experience are energy concentrations that need to be balanced through reflexology.

---

We are all connected, and we need to feel connected with each other. Touch is a way to establish and maintain this connection. In fact, it was discovered long ago that premature babies who were handled and stroked by their caretakers while in intensive care had a much greater survival rate than those who were not touched or not touched as often.

There's a difference between how I feel when I use my foot roller for reflexology and when my husband (my personal home-schooled reflexologist!) works on my feet. Subconsciously, you can convey messages through your touch. It's not only important to touch correctly for health, but you need to be aware of how to touch someone without making them uncomfortable.

Although I encourage you to practice reflexology on yourself, family members, and maybe a close friend with what you learn here, if you want to practice as a reflexologist, you will need to seek the appropriate training. Your instructor will be your best source for honing your hands-on skills. I always suggest getting a reflexology session from the instructor prior to signing up for their classes if possible, to see how you like what they do and how they feel to you. Good touch seems to be "handed down" from instructor to student. Becoming conscious of your touch will take some focus until you become skilled, and because it's key to a good reflexology session, it's important that I share some tips for you here.

# Keep Your Eyes on the Foot

Giving reflexology sessions can be a thoroughly relaxing experience, and it can be easy to drift off. Keeping your eyes on the feet helps you stay focused and diminishes the temptation to daydream while working on a person. This is especially true if you're working in a setting with a beautiful view out the window. If you gaze outside too long, you might find that you've worked your subject's descending colon for 15 minutes (not necessarily a good place to find yourself)!

Even if you know the areas to work on by feel, it still helps to keep your attention on the foot and the areas

> **Tip Toe**
>
> Avoid being distracted while you work. Remember, your goal is to help the person you're working on heal. They need your full attention to make this happen.

you're working on. You don't always have to stare directly at the foot or hand as you work, but keeping your gaze in that general direction is always a good idea. This gives the person you're working on confidence that you're paying attention to them, and it helps you stay on track as well.

Keeping both eyes and both hands always on the foot you're working on is a simple rule that will likely come naturally to you. One hand needs to be supporting the foot at all times, unless you're practicing techniques that use both hands at the same time. In the following section, I cover a couple two-handed techniques.

# Keep in Touch

When you first work on someone, you are basically introducing yourself (your hands) to their feet (or hands or ears, as the case may be). Think about that for a moment. When we meet another person, we generally shake their hand. This is usually truer of men than of women, and it's more common in the American tradition, but nevertheless it happens worldwide.

When we touch another person, information is exchanged through the touch. It's a subconscious process (although some of us make it a very conscious process) to judge someone by the feel of his or her handshake and the feel of their hand. Cold, sweaty, soft, or firm—all have different feels and mean different things to us.

## Don't Leave Me

When we make physical contact with another person, we also exchange energy. Our cells communicate with one another. It's important that you try to keep physical contact with the person's body throughout the reflexology session. When you're sending loving, healing thoughts to a person you're working on, their body will respond to you. You don't want to break that flow.

However, at times it's appropriate to break the flow. Your first concern should always be the person's comfort. Here are some subject "needs" when you may need to break contact:

- Needs to use the restroom. This urge is often stimulated by the reflexology work you're doing.

- Needs a tissue. Sometimes your partner releases emotional tears during a session or needs to blow his or her nose, which also can be brought on by your reflexology work.

◆ Needs a (or another) blanket. Sometimes a person gets chilly lying still while being worked on. Stop and provide them a blanket so they can fully enjoy the experience.

---

### Foot Note

Many of my clients fall asleep while I work on them. Some say they try to fight it so they don't miss any of the goodies, but they can't help themselves. One even took caffeine before he saw me because he loves the work I do so much he wanted to stay awake! He fell asleep anyway. I take it as a compliment that I have helped them relax thoroughly, that they have enough security with me to be able to let themselves fall asleep, and that I have gained their trust.

---

After making contact with the foot, if you break the contact completely, the body will respond to that change. It will keep your subject guessing at the subconscious level and keep them from relaxing fully. If you do have to break off, start up again gently. Keeping at least one hand on the foot at all times is a way of not breaking contact. If you use music and you need to replay a CD, for example, try to use a remote control. This allows you to maintain contact. If you're using lotion or oil and need to apply some to your hands, at least keep an elbow or a knee touching your subject's foot while you get more lotion.

Keeping contact during reflexology is like using the foot pedals on a piano. The foot pedals keep the chords flowing, and without them, the chords don't blend together. Each time you lift your fingers off the keys and before you strike some new chords, you hear a break in the flow. This is the same effect you get if you're "pounding on the piano" or when you're playing allegro pieces, such as ragtime music.

### Tip Toe

Even if the person does not recognize it consciously, when you connect with them, they get a sense of security that you're there. That can be a very comforting feeling. This continuous contact helps the person relax and maintain a peaceful state.

The touch you want to achieve with reflexology is like a flowing, smooth sonata. Keeping contact allows you to create a relaxing, healing experience in which each touch builds on the one before.

## Good for the Sole

By the way, this *contact-ual* agreement you make with the foot is not necessarily just benefiting the person you're working on! You also get the benefits of reflexology as you work on another person because your fingers are being stimulated as you work. When you use your thumb and fingertip techniques, your brain and sinus area reflexes are being stimulated simultaneously.

The reflexologist always seems to benefit from doing this work. For instance, my body always responds positively after I work on clients all day. I feel energized, clear, and more alert, although I also feel very relaxed. I sleep better, and my appetite is suppressed (meaning I don't feel the need to overindulge in foods that are not best for me). Many times people comment afterward that I have a glow or my eyes look clear and bright after a day of giving reflexology.

Reflexology not only gives the practitioner some physical benefits, but it may also be good for the soul. So what I'm really saying is "What's good for your sole is good for my soul."

# Happiness Runs in a Circular Motion

So now we've learned about the energy exchanged when you touch someone. Maybe that's why it feels nicer to have another work on you versus doing all your own reflexology work on yourself. Maybe somehow our bodies exchange energy and balance each other out when we touch. In any case, let's now take a look at some more wonderful techniques you can use on your partner to induce relaxation. The following moves are all rotations and circular movements and are like warm-up exercises for your body.

Circular motions are used in a roundabout way in reflexology. One of the first things you can do to loosen up the foot and begin relaxation is called an *ankle rotation*. You can rotate the foot on its ankle in a few ways. I've included some photos to show you how to hold the foot to perform these rotations. Remember that the foot does not revolve around you—you revolve around the foot!

## Ankle Rotation

The first and easiest way to perform an ankle rotation is the following:

◆ With one hand, cup the whole ankle like you're holding a large, hardboiled egg in your hand. Support it, but don't squeeze too hard.

◆ With the other hand, grasp the ball (padding) of the foot. Lay your four fingers across the top part of the foot just below the toes with your thumb across the ball of the foot, just below the toes.

◆ With the hand that's grasping the top of the foot, gently rotate the foot in a counterclockwise direction.

◆ Go s-l-o-w-l-y and stretch the foot as far as is comfortable for your partner.

◆ Rotate the foot three times counterclockwise and then three times clockwise.

Usually this feels so good to the person receiving the ankle rotation that if you're not stretching it far enough, they'll "help" you by rotating the foot themselves. Encourage them to relax if that happens, and give them a wider stretch (circle).

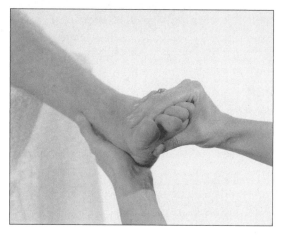

*Rotate the foot three times in a counterclockwise direction and then three times in a clockwise direction. Stretch the foot as far as is comfortable.*

## Toe-Spreading Rotation

If the person you're working on has toes with sufficient space between them, you can use another method for ankle rotation. The basic movements are the same, but the way you grasp the foot is different. Place your four fingers between the four spaces of the toes and then rotate.

This method gives the upper lymph nodes a little stimulation and stretches the toes a bit. If you find yourself struggling to get your fingers between the toes, bypass this method. It will probably be uncomfortable for your subject. Over time, reflexology sessions will help the toes gain more flexibility, and you can try this method in subsequent sessions.

*Use this method of ankle rotation only if toe space permits!*

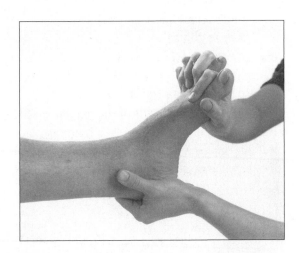

## Menstrual Relief Rotation

You can use another form of foot/ankle rotation for relaxation and for stimulating the fallopian tube/spermatic cord/pelvic region (see Chapter 15). This is great for a stiff lower back or hips and for menstrual trouble or pain.

◆ Grasp the top side of the ankle from the front, with the webbing between your thumb and index finger pressing against the fallopian tube/spermatic cord region. In this position, if your fingers are long enough, they'll fall just about where the ovary/testes and uterus/prostate points are located on either side of the heel, which will stimulate these areas at the same time.

♦ With your other hand, grasp the top of the foot with the palm of your hand against the tops of the toes and your fingers overlapping the bottoms of the toes, kind of like you would grasp this book as you're pulling it off your shelf to read again! Use this hand to rotate the foot.

♦ When you get to the top of the foot in your rotation, rotate the foot into the webbing of the grasped hand to apply pressure to the fallopian tube/ spermatic cord reflex.

Rotate the ankle three times in each direction using this method.

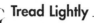 **Tread Lightly** _____

Reflexology should not be used in place of moving your body daily. Although reflexology is wonderful and stimulates the whole body, the feet were made for walking. Walking is one of the best exercises you can perform for the overall health of your body and your feet!

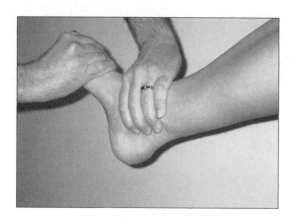

*This method is good if the person is having menstrual or prostate difficulties or has a sore lower back or hips.*

# Finger and Thumb Rolls

Other circular motions involve using the finger and thumb techniques you learned in Chapter 5 to roll them on the reflex points. For instance, the sex organ reflex points are excellent points to utilize finger and thumb rotations.

You can stimulate the ovary/testes point with the thumb or finger. This spot is on the outside of each foot about halfway between the ankle and heel (see Chapter 15). Find the area, apply firm pressure, and rotate your thumb or finger on this spot without lifting it. Be sure you're not just rotating your finger around the surface of the skin. You can try this technique on yourself easily by bringing up your foot, as shown in the following photos.

For the uterus/prostate point, which is in approximately the same location on the inside of the foot, you can perform the same technique using your fingers or thumb. Find the spot, press in, rotate three times counterclockwise, and then rotate three times clockwise. You can also just press the point, hold it for three seconds, release, and repeat two more times. Both of these areas will more than likely be tender on most people. I find they are more tender on females the closer they are to their time of the month or near their *ovulation*. This spot is also great for a woman experiencing menstrual cramps.

## def•i•ni•tion

**Ovulation** is the time in a woman's menstrual cycle when the ovaries produce an egg and deliver it to the uterus to be (sometimes) fertilized. This process is controlled by the hormones secreted by the pituitary gland.

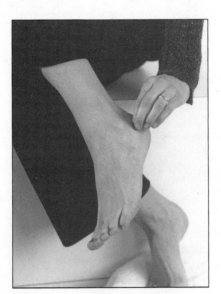 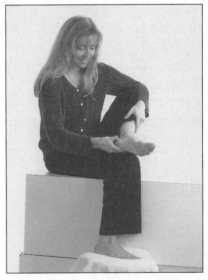

*You can use this technique on yourself easily or on others. Press in and rotate on each spot three times counterclockwise and then three times clockwise.*

## Tootsie Rolls and Rotating Toes

Another rotating move that will get you rockin' and rollin' is what my teacher nicknamed "tootsie rolls." Tootsie rolls are another good warm-up technique to help the entire body relax and also stimulates the sinuses to release congestion. Tootsie rolls and rotating toes can both be used to get a reflexology session started.

Tootsie rolls are just like miniature yummies (see Chapter 4). To make tootsie rolls, take each toe between the palm side of your fingers. Keeping your fingers straight, move each hand in an opposite direction and "roll" the toe between them. Do you remember playing with Play-Doh when you were a child and making snakes? You roll a blob of clay between your hands until it is a long, snakelike piece. This is how tootsie rolls are performed!

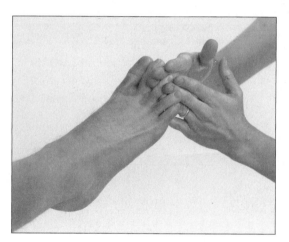

*Pretend you're making clay snakes while rolling each toe.*

Another related—and fantastically relaxing—technique involves rolling or rotating each toe. Sometimes this puts the recipient to sleep right off the bat. For this technique, use one hand to support the ball of the foot at the base of the toes. Hold this part firmly. Grasp the baby toe at the tip, and slowly rotate the toe three times counterclockwise and then three times clockwise. You can liken this toe-rotating movement to mixing a Barbie-size bowl of cake batter! If you remember, this technique is included in your 10-minute quickie routine in Chapter 4. Do this to each toe. Rotate the toes in a circle as wide as you can without causing your partner any discomfort.

Remember, the reflex for the head and neck is the large toe. Therefore, rotating the large toe is like doing neck rolls. If you feel crunchies as you rotate the large toe, this is a good indication of a stiff neck or that a neck vertebra is out of alignment. Usually after the rotations, most if not all of the crunchies and crackling disappear. The rotation helps loosen up the neck and may help it back into alignment. Sometimes the receiver will feel pulsating, goose bumps, or a crawling sensation in the scalp or neck when you rotate their toes—especially the large toe.

After rotating each toe, you can gently pull upward on the toes. Sometimes the toe "pops" or cracks. This might surprise the subject, but it should feel very good to them. This usually happens because the tootsie rolls and toe rotations loosened up the toes. If the toe was misaligned at all, a gentle pull sometimes causes the toe to go back into alignment. Do not do this forcefully. A gentle pull will most likely do the trick.

---

### Foot Note

In my experience, reflexology seems to be an effective pain-relieving session for people with arthritic feet. One such client gained great relief that lasted for days after my sessions. At times, I accidentally would "pop" his toes, which caused him to jump. Afterward, he would tell me how much better the "popped" toes felt, and he began requesting that I do it every time.

---

# No Pinching Allowed

When practicing reflexology, be careful not to pinch or pull the skin. Reflexology involves techniques that apply pressure, rotations, and gentle but firm movements. You don't want to pull, rub, or pinch the skin.

To avoid this, when you're moving up the foot or hand with finger or thumb walking, be sure you lift your fingers up just enough to let the skin fall back into place. Or use some talcum powder or a dab of oil to help your fingers slide over the skin. This is especially helpful when the person you're working on has very dry or scaly skin.

Touch is important, but *how* you touch is even more important. You need to learn to be aware of every way your body is interacting with another. This is true for all types of bodywork. You need to be especially aware of what your other hand is doing when you're working on the body with one hand. For instance, when thumb walking across the lung reflexes, be sure the fingernails of your supporting hand are not digging into the skin.

*Bedside manner*, a term used to describe how doctors interact with their patients, fits what I'm talking about here. You need to have a good bedside manner to be an effective reflexologist. But a good bedside manner in reflexology is more than just acting and behaving professionally.

**def•i•ni•tion**

**Bedside manner** is a term used to describe how a doctor behaves in front of or toward a patient. Reflexologists also need to develop a good bedside manner to make the recipient feel comfortable, at ease, relaxed, and well cared for.

First of all, as you already know, keep your fingernails trimmed. Second, don't forget about warming your hands before you touch someone! Rub your hands vigorously together or keep a warmed towel nearby to heat up your hands before you start working on someone. This is part of good bedside manner, too.

Additionally, be aware of *both* hands and other things that might touch your subject. For example, you probably want to take off any bulky jewelry that could interfere with a session. Your friend won't like it if you get his leg or toe hairs stuck in your watchband! Ouch!

**Tip Toe**

Before working on a partner, always ask them to remove all their jewelry. It's easier to work on a foot or hand with no jewelry, but some folks might not be willing to take off their wedding ring. Be sensitive to the issue; you can always work around it if you must!

Because you are so focused on the techniques you're doing with one hand, don't become oblivious to the fact that a diamond from your wedding ring is sticking into your subject's foot!

# Injured Areas: Don't Go There

The first rule of being a reflexologist—before you even get started with all these fun techniques—is to make a visual observation of the foot. You need to look for injuries, cuts, and other ailments, because you don't want to work directly on any such injured areas. It's also important not to work on someone else if you have any contagious conditions yourself, such as fungus growths. (Athlete's foot, for example, is a fungus that can grow on the hands, too.) If you have a contagious ailment, it may spread through an open cut on your hand, so wait until you're over it before you work on others. Some professional reflexologists have worn sterile rubber gloves to work on folks for the protection of both the client and the reflexologist, although this is rare. Of course, you'll learn all this in your training as a professional reflexologist, but I wanted to mention it so you don't wind up sharing more than you want to with the family members and close friends you do practice on!

## Edema: Got the Dropsy's?

One *contraindication* for reflexology is working on a person with edema in the feet. Many of us hold excess water occasionally, especially women before menstruation. This type of edema is referred to as subcutaneous edema and is not very serious. Keeping the legs elevated usually corrects this condition.

### def•i•ni•tion

A **contraindication** is any factor that makes it unwise to pursue a certain line of treatment. For example, you would not give a massage to a person with severe sunburn!

However, edema is an excessive accumulation of fluid in the body tissues. This condition is serious because there may be collections of fluid in the chest cavity and in the air spaces of the lung (pulmonary edema) causing severe chest congestion.

Edema may result from heart or kidney failure, cirrhosis of the liver, allergies, or drugs. If you have severe swelling of the legs, feet, and ankles, do not work on these areas directly. Instead, work on the hands, and get to your medical physician immediately.

## Varicose Veins: Varying the Treatment

Most of us are familiar with varicose veins. Varicose veins are long and distended veins and can appear purple when you see them just under the surface of the skin, most commonly in the superficial veins of the legs.

There may be an inherited tendency to varicose veins, but it is aggravated or can be caused by an obstruction of blood flow in the body.

If you have knotty, irregular-shaped, or dilated varicose veins, reflexology would be contraindicated. You should not reflex these areas if you have them or if you are working on someone with such veins. You can work the corresponding part instead, but do not work directly on the area. If you see an injured foot, you always have the option to work on the corresponding hand instead, and vice versa. For instance, when you find irregular varicose veins in the left foot, you can gently work the left hand instead.

**Tread Lightly**

The tiny broken blood vessels you sometimes see on your feet may indicate a problem with the circulatory system in general, and you should consider seeing a holistic health practitioner to help you strengthen your circulatory system nutritionally.

Some other contraindications you should be aware of are listed in the following table.

## Reflexology Contraindications

| Foot Condition | Why You Shouldn't Go There | What to Do Instead |
|---|---|---|
| Knotty, irregular-shaped, or dilated varicose veins | Reflexology may put too much pressure on these veins and break more blood vessels | Work around these areas, or work the corresponding part instead (i.e., for varicose veins in left calf, work left forearm) |
| Severe swelling of the foot (edema) | Could mean insufficient blood flow and blockage of lymph system or heart disease | Refer this person to their doctor immediately and work the hands |

*continues*

## Reflexology Contraindications (continued)

| Foot Condition | Why You Shouldn't Go There | What to Do Instead |
|---|---|---|
| Fractures, surgeries, or sprains | Could interfere with healing | Do not work directly on; work the same side corresponding part (i.e., wrist fracture on left wrist; work left ankle instead) |
| Contagious diseases or infections in either the subject or practitioner | For the health protection of all involved | Wait until the infection has cleared |
| Open wounds | Health protection | Wait until the wound has healed (to facilitate healing, work the corresponding part far removed from open wound) |
| Ingrown toenails or corns | Can cause pain | Don't work directly on these areas; refer to podiatrist |
| Gout | Could raise blood pressure and cause discomfort | Work lightly and discuss the contraindication with the subject; do not work on swollen area, instead work on kidneys, adrenals, and pancreas reflexes; refer to herbalist or holistic nutritionist for nutritional support |

Contraindications are warning signs. When you see these things, use caution or do not work on someone, and always refer your friends and family members to their physician for any medical necessities.

Reflexology relies on the interconnectedness of the whole body and the energy zones (zone therapy) that run along our body channels (see Chapter 1). Knowing this, when dealing with a contraindication, you can still work on an area of the body that runs along the same energy lines, but on a different part of the body.

Say, for instance, you broke or sprained your right ankle. Your first goal will probably be to get someone to take you to the doctor for treatment. In the meantime, you can apply ice to the ankle (first aid) and then you can begin "reflexing" your right wrist to facilitate healing and possibly alleviate the pain in your ankle. During the healing process, working the corresponding wrist will help your ankle heal. Don't forget to work the other wrist as well, because the body needs balance. But it's okay to work the corresponding wrist more, because that's the side of the body that requires more energy for healing.

Overall, be aware of both of your hands, keep in contact, and look for contraindications, and you will be on the road to becoming a very effective and appreciated reflexologist!

## The Least You Need to Know

- Keep your eyes on the areas you're working on to stay focused and to gain your subject's confidence.

- Maintain physical contact throughout a reflexology session to help your partner relax more thoroughly and keep the energy exchange flowing.

- Be aware of both hands when performing reflexology. Be sure not to pinch the skin, and don't forget to remove your jewelry and have your partner remove theirs.

- Before performing any reflexology techniques, first observe the area you're going to work on. If you observe any injuries, cuts, ulcers, or other ailments, do not work there.

- Be aware of the contraindications to reflexology, and be sure to allow for them before you begin.

# Chapter 7

# Third Time's a Charm

## In This Chapter

- Discover the mystery of the number three
- Learn why reflexologists do everything three times
- Understand how reflexology works on more than the physical level
- Find out how to use your knuckles—and how not to
- Learn some gripping, stretching, and twisting techniques

Well, now you know about all the rolling and rotating techniques and you find yourself relaxed and looking forward to more. Have you wondered why I keep instructing you to do each move and rotation three times? Well, even if you haven't wondered, I give you some reasons in this chapter! After some philosophical talk on the mystery of threes, I introduce you to three new reflexology techniques you can use three times each to make you feel three times as good!

# Doing the Math

The meaning of numbers underlies everything in our lives. Certain meanings are attached to numbers that go deep into humanity's early beginnings, as taught in the Jewish Kabbalah. Have you ever given any thought to how we use numbers in everything we do? Our modern world couldn't exist as we know it without the framework numbers give us. Could our whole reality be a giant math problem? Imagine that!

For instance, you're now reading Chapter 7 and are on a certain page number and have been reading for a certain number of minutes or hours. You live at an address with numbers in it, and you need numbers to make a phone call. You have some sort of identifying number, such as a Social Security number or a tax ID number. Names can even be broken down into numbers and then analyzed (as in numerology).

Think about trying to buy this book without the use of numbers in the transaction! You'd never make it, would you? You find this book in a bookstore with a certain address, in a certain numbered aisle, on a certain row number, with a certain price on it. Most places charge you a certain percentage in tax, and you need a certain amount of money to pay for it.

Reflexology is no exception. Most of your sessions will be timed to last a certain number of minutes, and if you're charging for your sessions, you'll charge a certain amount of money. Furthermore, you usually work with 2 feet and 10 toes. Reflexologists take this one step further, though, and use a particular number as a basis for their work: the number three.

# The Mystery of Threes

Why is it that the third time's a charm? And why were there three little pigs, three bears, three blind mice, and Three Stooges? Why do they say bad things happen in threes? Why do I only get three wishes and have to knock three times on the ceiling if I want you?

The mystery of threes has not yet been unlocked, although the number's roots can be linked to Christianity and the Trinity of Father, Son, and Holy Spirit. But most of us haven't really given much thought to the mystery of the number three. I like three because it always gives us a middle ground:

- Small, medium, large

- Past, present, future

- Short, average, tall

- Left, middle, right

You can always choose the middle ground if you're unsure, but only if you have three choices to begin with. I like the middle choice for simple decisions because it can take the stress out of the decision-making process. The medium size is what the "average" person requires. People choose the middle ground for peaceful negotiations.

Besides, the middle choice seems to be more balanced. Not that there's no validity in extremes, but the middle is usually where most of us function. Three may be a number that forces one to integrate. I see it as a peaceful number. There is black, and there is white. Both extremes are easy to understand because both are clear-cut. However, dealing with someone who is purely black or white in their thinking leaves no room for compromise. Many can live with some things in the gray areas.

---

### Foot Note

*Numerology* is the study of numbers and their synchronicity in our lives. In numerology, the three energy symbolizes communication, creativity, humor, and the integration of the physical, mental, and spiritual. This is just a generalization to introduce you to the concept. Consult *The Complete Idiot's Guide to Astrology*, now in its third edition (Alpha Books, 2003), and *The Complete Idiot's Guide to Numerology*, now in its second edition (Alpha Books, 2004), for more details on this fun subject.

---

For the purpose of reflexology, you'll want to practice your techniques with the number three in mind. Each technique should be performed three times. For example, if you're doing rotations, rotate the foot three times in each direction. When you're utilizing pressure points, press and hold three seconds and then release. Repeat for a total of three times.

After you're a trained reflexologist in practice, or even if you're just trying to convince your spouse that reflexology works, you should encourage subjects to try out a reflexology session at least three times—not too far apart, say once a week for 3 weeks—to see the real benefits. Then they should continue regular sessions for a minimum of 3 months for lasting effects.

# Body, Mind, and Sole

Physically, reflexology is beneficial both to the recipient and to the person who administers it. But it goes even further than just stimulating our mutual reflex points. It can also have an effect on all three parts of us: our body, our mind, and our spirit.

I talked earlier about the importance of touch and the energy that's exchanged. Touch can make a person's body feel good, and it can also positively affect the mind. When you're being touched in a healing way, it can trigger a self-love response in your subconscious. The fact that you have allowed someone to care for you and help you heal means you have taken time out to care for yourself. Self-love can have a positive effect on the immune system as well.

Why does reflexology work on the practitioner's spirit? Well, when you're taking care of someone with reflexology, it's usually because you have an inner urge to help people or a calling to heal. I believe this inner urging or calling comes from the spirit or soul. Anything you feel in your heart and soul should be expressed.

The heart is the seat of the soul and cannot give you messages to do harm. Of course, the heart/soul's desire always needs to be tempered with the intellect. But there should be no denying your deep calling to do what you are meant to do. Your heart will communicate with you.

# Knead Me, Heel Me

Although it's a cute pun, reflexologists really don't *knead* anybody! Kneading is really more a term for kneading dough, and massage therapists use this term loosely as a play on words for their work.

Reflexologists use their hands as their tools to work on their subjects. Some professional reflexologists employ tools in their practice as well. But for the most part, reflexologists' hands are their biggest assets. Some professional reflexology organizations prohibit the use of knuckles during reflexology sessions because they consider the use of knuckles a tool or because they believe knuckles can exert too much pressure on a client.

If you prefer deep work and want to work on yourself at home, feel free to use your knuckles, foot rollers, or any other tools you want as long as you use common sense to determine what's helpful for you and what might hurt you. You know your pain tolerance better than anyone.

## Knuckling In

Some of the self-help techniques you can apply in reflexology can be done with your knuckles. The knuckles can exert much more pressure than your thumb or fingers alone and should be used carefully if you choose to use them on a family member.

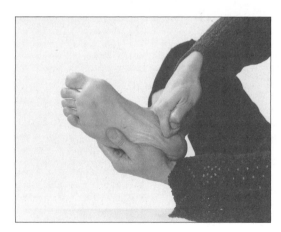

*Knuckle walking. This is a great method if you have hemorrhoids or hip, back, or pelvic troubles.*

I especially like to use my knuckles to work my heel. The heel represents the lower pelvic region and hip area. To use this method, you can perform a kind of knuckle walk with the middle knuckle of your pointer finger of one hand while you support the ankle with the other.

Use your knuckle and walk across from one side of the heel to the other. This technique really helps stimulate the circulation to the various areas. This is a great therapy if you have hip pain, lower back pain, pelvic troubles, and/or hemorrhoids.

# I Can Breathe Clearly Now

Another method that utilizes the knuckles is great for the respiratory system, chest, lungs, bronchial tubes, diaphragm, back, and neck. To use this technique, follow these steps:

♦ Support the metatarsal bones (top of the foot) with one hand.

♦ Bend all four fingers in toward the palm of the other hand, but don't touch your fingertips to your palm as you would with a fist.

♦ Gently press your knuckles into the padding of the foot below the toes with one hand as you support the top of the foot with the other.

♦ Hold for 3 seconds, release, and then repeat two more times.

## Tip Toe

In general, working a certain reflex area three times helps give balance to your reflexology sessions. You can always go back after you've reflexed everything three times and work more on the tender spots; those are the areas that usually require the most work.

Take a look at the following photo to see this technique in action.

*This technique can aid the chest, lungs, bronchial tubes, diaphragm, back, and neck. Hold for 3 seconds, release, and then repeat two more times.*

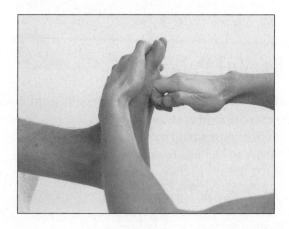

# Up, Down, and Back Again

Another great move that comes in threes is walking up the spine reflex. In earlier chapters, you learned that the spine gives us structure, but it also houses the main nervous system cables, putting it in both the structural system and nervous system categories. Working this reflex is wonderfully relaxing, and although this reflex can be worked indefinitely, you should remember to cover it at least three times.

Thumb walking is great for walking up the spine reflex. Start at the bottom of the heel with your thumb and walk all the way to the top of the large toe. When you get to the top, turn around and walk back down again. Walk up one more time and then you're through. Whomever you are working on will be peacefully relaxed after this technique. You can always get your three times in if you remember to work up, down, and back again.

> **Tread Lightly**
>
> Never push or shove the foot in any direction it doesn't want to go, nor farther than what's comfortable for your subject.

This technique can be used to work the urinary system as well. You can start at the bladder reflex area, thumb walk up over the ureter, and on to the kidney. Then come back down from the kidney, down along the ureter tube reflex to the bladder, and then one more time back up to complete the cycle.

# Ready? Relax!

It's always a good idea to loosen up the feet before stimulating reflex points. The three stretching techniques in this section—"Bend and Stretch" (stretching out the feet to get them warmed up for reflexology), "Twist and Shout" (a spinal twist you'll be sure to shout about), and "Wringing Out the Stress" (another squeezing and wringing technique for relaxation)—help you relax your legs, feet, and entire body, which, in turn, helps you get more benefit out of the session.

> **Tread Lightly**
>
> Be careful not to pull or tug on the hair on the legs whenever you're practicing techniques on the lower part of a person's leg.

## Bend and Stretch

The first stretching technique we're going to learn helps the person's whole leg relax, especially the back of the calves and hamstrings. This technique also gets the feet and ankles loosened up, helps increase circulation, and prepares the person to respond better to reflexology. Here's how to do it:

 ◆ First, cup the underside of the heel in the palm of your hand. This is the same grip you used to rotate the feet in the last chapter.

 ◆ Next, grasp the top part of the foot with your other hand. This is also the same grip you used with the rotation techniques. Be sure not to squeeze the foot on top and pinch the skin! The grip should come naturally. Your hand will grasp the outside of the foot around the ball with your thumb resting on the inside padding of the ball of the foot.

 ◆ Pull the top part of the foot toward you slowly as far as is comfortable for the person. Hold for a moment to allow the muscles to relax into the stretch. Instruct the person to exhale as you stretch the muscle.

 ◆ Do not grip the heel tightly. Let it move naturally with the stretch.

 ◆ Then push the top of the foot gently back toward the person as far as it will go. You can use the heel of your hand to push at the pad of the ball of the foot to get a good stretch. Hold this position momentarily. You do not want to hold this position for too long, as it could cause the foot to cramp.

 ◆ If the foot seems very stiff, first try one of the rotating techniques from Chapter 6 or a yummy and then try this stretch again. If the person has a lot of tension in their legs, this stretch helps them be more flexible.

And I bet you'll never guess how many times you should do this stretch. You're right—repeat this procedure three times back and forth on each foot.

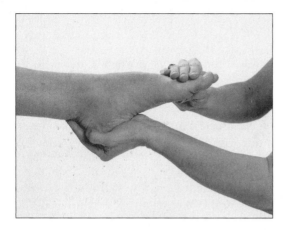

*Stretching technique step 1: stretch the foot forward (toward you) and hold momentarily to let the muscles ease into the stretch.*

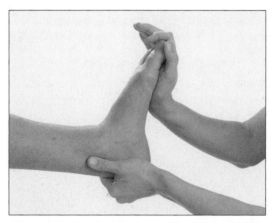

*Stretching technique step 2: push the foot gently back (toward the subject's knee) and hold only briefly to avoid causing a cramp.*

---

### Foot Note

You can adapt the bend and stretch technique to suit the four directions if you'd rather. After stretching the foot to the front and back, stretch the foot to the inside (medially), while steadying the heel. Then move the foot laterally as far as the recipient will allow. Do each stretch the same number of times. You have now done the four directions. Now rotate the foot in a circular motion counterclockwise, then clockwise.

---

## Twist and Shout

Next is a twisting technique used by practitioners to relax the body. It can even have an effect on the alignment of the spinal column. In fact, I call it a "spinal twist."

To perform this technique, take a look at the next two photos and follow these steps:

♦ Grasp the top (dorsal side) of the foot, just below the ankle. Both of your hands should grasp the foot firmly, and your thumbs should be resting on the inside sole of the foot, just above the heel.

♦ Begin moving the hand closest to the toes in short, firm motions, twisting the foot from side to side. Firmly hold the rest of the foot with the other hand.

♦ After a few "twists," move both hands slightly up (toward the toes) and twist again. You can work this motion all the way up to the top part of the toes.

♦ When you get to the toes, you can begin the same motion back down toward the heel again.

♦ And—you guessed it—next you go back up one more time for a total of three times on each foot.

This technique helps relax all the back muscles and is extremely rejuvenating to the entire body.

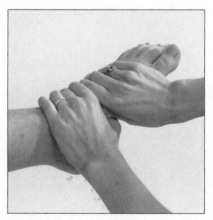 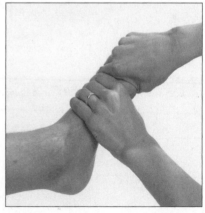

*Spinal twist starting point: begin at the heel and work your way up, slightly, twisting the hand closest to the toes. This works the entire spinal region.*

*Spinal twist ending point: when you get to the toes, work your way back down to the heel and then go back up one more time.*

**Tip Toe** _____

When you're squeezing and stretching the foot in these and other techniques, keep in mind it's the same as squeezing the whole body—kind of like hugging! When you hug someone, squeezing too tight is uncomfortable, but if you squeeze too lightly you appear insincere. So go for the third choice, which is *just right!*

## Wringing Out the Stress

The third relaxation technique involves wringing the foot. This opens up the lymphatic system and is good for any type of chest congestion. For this technique, imagine the foot is a sopping-wet towel or mop. Your job is to wring out the excess water. (Just remember that you don't need to squeeze it dry!) Does the wringing technique ring a bell with you? It should. It's similar to the spinal twist, but is slower and involves more squeezing.

To perform this technique:

♦ Lay your fingers across the top part of the foot.

♦ Place your hands one just above the other, reaching in from opposite sides of the foot. In this position your thumbs will be on the plantar (underside) surface of the foot.

♦ Gently squeeze both hands as you slightly turn each hand in opposite directions.

♦ Move slowly upward and repeat two more times, moving from the ankle on up to the toes each time.

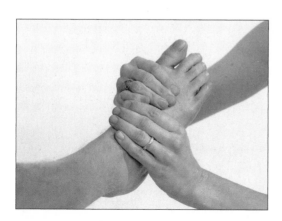

*Wringing the foot: pretend the foot is a sopping-wet towel and you're wringing out the excess water. Be careful not to pull the skin on this one!*

I hope these three new techniques—stretching, twisting, and wringing—bring you and your partner a great deal of pleasure, and that pleasure is experienced threefold by making you healthy, wealthy, and wise!

## The Least You Need to Know

◆ The number three symbolizes the integration of the physical, mental, and spiritual aspects of a person, which is a goal of reflexology. Reflexology not only works on the physical body, but can have far-reaching, positive effects on the mind and spirit.

◆ In reflexology, you practice each technique three times on each foot or hand.

◆ You can use your knuckles if your thumbs are tired. The knuckles can be used to exert more pressure along tougher areas, such as the heel.

◆ Twisting, wringing, and stretching the feet are all great techniques for bringing more flexibility to the legs, feet, and ankles and can enhance a reflexology session by helping the person relax.

# The Body Systems: Mapping It Out

What's the best way to your partner's heart? It just might be through his feet! Not only can you create goodwill by practicing reflexology on your partner's feet, but you may actually help prevent heart-related troubles!

Within Part 3 lie the secrets to reflexology—how reflex points in the feet and hands affect the rest of the body. Now we get to see what those body parts correspond to on the foot map. Here we take a body-systems approach to understanding the body's functions. Classifying major organs into basic systems is a simple way to get to know yourself from the inside out.

I think you'll enjoy this fun look into your own body. And remember, a journey of a thousand miles begins with the first step.

# Chapter 8

# In Your Defense:
# The Immune System

## In This Chapter

- ◆ Learn the importance of the immune system
- ◆ Understand some of the immune system's organs
- ◆ See how the immune system affects your health
- ◆ Locate the immune reflex points on the feet and hands

There were three rabbits, the first one named Foot, the second, Foot Foot, and the third, Foot Foot Foot. One day Foot was feeling sick, so Foot Foot and Foot Foot Foot took Foot to a doctor, who told Foot Foot and Foot Foot Foot that Foot was going to die. Sure enough, Foot died. The following month, Foot Foot felt ill. So Foot Foot Foot packed up Foot Foot and took him to a different doctor. The new doctor gave Foot Foot a thorough examination and told Foot Foot Foot that Foot Foot was very ill. Foot Foot Foot became hysterical: "You've got to save him, doctor. We already have one Foot in the grave."

The moral of this corny joke is that the proper functioning of the immune system is key to your health and your life! It's like your own internal army fighting off invaders, viruses, bacteria, and parasites in a battle to maintain your body's right to enjoy health. Now get ready to be all you can be and join me for a look at your personal armed forces.

# Granting Immunity

How do you know when your immune system is not up to par? Here are some clues: recurring infections, frequent colds or illness, slow-healing wounds, and frequent viral breakouts. Reflexology can play a key role in keeping your immune system strong and functioning properly.

Along with a good diet, supplements, and a positive mental attitude, reflexology is another round of ammunition for your immune system's army of soldiers to utilize. If you're sick or fighting off an infection or any type of disease, strengthening your immune system is the best thing you can do to help yourself.

Many, many organs affect your immune system and are responsible for killing bugs and evicting invaders. I'm only going to talk about the primary functions of each of the body systems and their principal organs for simplicity.

# A Note on Understanding the Diagrams

Before reading further, you might want to glance at the figures that follow to get a general idea of the immune system's organs and the corresponding areas on the foot and hand. You'll see the same basic foot and hand charts throughout the book, showing different reflex locations as appropriate per each chapter. Unless otherwise indicated, what you see is always the bottom of the foot and the palm of the hand.

I've also included two lines in the diagrams. These are the hip line and the diaphragm line, which give you a reference point and a way to divide the feet and/or hands into three sections. You can visualize anything above the diaphragm line as being reflexes to your upper body (from your diaphragm up). The middle section covers reflexes predominately in the trunk area, and the hip line is basically where your hip reflexes are. Below the hip line on the sole of the foot, there are very few reflexes. Sometimes you'll see the waist line through the middle of the foot; again, this is just for your orientation and happens to be the reflex area for your waist, too.

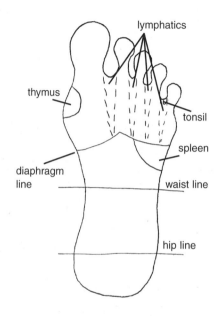

*The foot reflex points for the immune system, shown on the left foot. The lymphatic, tonsil, and thymus reflexes are also located on the right foot.*

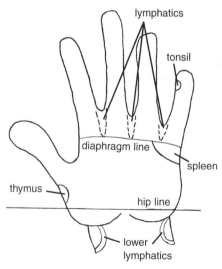

*The left hand reflex points for the immune system. The lymphatics, tonsil, and thymus reflexes are also located in the same areas on the right hand.*

I usually use the palm of the left hand for the diagrams. You can see this if you hold your left hand in front of you with your palm turned toward you. I also primarily use a left foot for most of the diagrams. This view would be the view of the bottom of the foot if a person was lying down and you were sitting at their feet, looking at the sole of their foot.

For simplicity and clarity, I've only used the left hand or left foot throughout these pages; however, this *does not* mean that the same reflexes are not located on the same areas on the opposite foot or hand. For the most part, our body has a pair of everything: a pair of lungs, eyes, ears, kidneys, and so on. Just as this is true in the body, it's true for the reflex areas on the foot. Where there is only one organ on one side of the body or where the reflexes differ from one hand or foot to the other, I've included both hands or feet in the diagrams. Don't worry—I won't lose you.

**Tip Toe**

Your body is a whole unit, so you should always work on both feet or both hands to get balanced results.

Feel free to press gently on the reflex points and get familiar with these organs and reflex spots as I refer to them along the way. Most points you should try to press in deeper until you do find a little tenderness. Then you know you're accessing the reflex. You'll notice that some reflexes are deeper than others, depending on the health or balance of the corresponding organ at the time. You can work on these immune system areas anytime you're not feeling well, and it can speed your recovery time.

---

**Foot Note**

Although reflexologists all agree that reflexology works, not all reflexology charts are identical. You will see slight differences in almost every chart you find. This book has simplified the reflexology charts to cover the basics and focus primarily on the soles and palms. After you get the basics down, be sure to obtain a nice, detailed wall chart for yourself. It's also a good idea to carry a laminated pocket card with you for reference when you're away from home.

---

# Your Keen Spleen

Your spleen is an organ located on the left side of the trunk of your body just under your diaphragm (or lower-left rib), above the waist, to the left of the stomach. The spleen reflex on the foot is also located on the left foot, just under the ball of the foot toward the outside edge of the foot's side, as shown in the previous figure.

The main spleen reflex point on the hand is also on the left hand, below the padding of the pinky finger, as shown in the previous figure.

The spleen is responsible for storing and filtering old and damaged blood cells, storing iron, manufacturing protective antibodies, and ridding the body of bacteria. The spleen also aids your body in producing new hemoglobin from old cells. Cool recycling program, eh?

> **Foot Note**
>
> If the spleen has been removed, the liver takes over the duties of the missing spleen. The liver is the overachieving organ in the body, performing hundreds of functions. (The liver is covered in Chapter 9 with the digestive and intestinal system.)

The spleen is actually a lymphatic gland and is the largest mass of lymphatic tissue in the body. It also manufactures protective antibodies, which go out on the battlefield and kill off offending invaders trying to stir up trouble in your system. Antibodies are, therefore, an important element in the functioning of your immune system.

Because the spleen has a big job in recycling the parts of old, worn-out cells and using their donated parts for the manufacture of new blood cells, the spleen is important to work on when there is indication of anemia in the body. Anemia is basically a very low red blood count. Symptoms include fatigue, a pale look to the skin, and poor resistance to infection. The spleen reflex point is an important spot to stimulate on the foot when one has symptoms of severe fatigue or a lowered immune response.

# Lymph-ing Along

The *lymphatic system* is a network of small, transparent lymph vessels that parallel the vein and artery pathways. The lymph vessels collect fluid that seeps through the blood vessel walls and then return the fluid back into the bloodstream after a filtering process. The lymph system includes the tonsils and all the lymph nodes throughout the body.

Many of our lymph nodes are located in the upper body around the neck and under the armpits. Because the brain is the ruler of the body, there are numerous lymph glands in the neck to protect the brain from infection—kind of like knights guarding the king's castle.

The lymph glands are responsible for producing white blood cells that destroy infection. These glands also absorb foreign invaders and kill them. You can experience the battle of your body working for you when you have a cold or sore throat and your neck glands are swollen.

This is your body's defense system working hard to fight off infection locally so the infection won't spread to the rest of your body.

**Tip Toe**

Besides jumping type exercises, the best way to clean the lymphatic system is with reflexology. Reflexology gets the entire circulatory system moving again, which also helps the lymph flow.

The reflex areas for the lymphatic system can be found between the webbing of the toes of both feet. The webbing between the first and second toes is equivalent to the neck area lymph glands. The webbing between the second and third and the third and fourth toes are the upper body and chest area in general. The webbing between the fourth and fifth toes is the reflex area for the armpits.

Squeezing all the webbing between all the metatarsals effectively works the entire lymph system. You can also thumb and finger nibble on the areas above each ankle (just above the fallopian tube reflexes) in an X across the front of the ankle to get more of the lower lymphatics, such as the groin area. The lower groin lymphs are also worked automatically when you do the ankle rotation techniques.

In the hands, the upper lymphatic reflexes are also located within the webbing between the fingers.

# Thymus Be Strong

Lymph-ing right along now, let's address another important component of the immune system. Many people believe that the *thymus gland* (pronounced *thigh-mus*) is really the seat of our immune system. This pinkish-gray, two-lobed organ is located in the chest cavity behind the upper sternum, below the thyroid. Basically, it sits right at the base of the neck.

The thymus reflex area on the foot is the medial edge of each big toe. (The medial side means the inside; it's the side of the foot that touches your other foot when you're standing with your feet together.) The point actually covers about 1 inch and is located almost in the middle of the joint halfway between the top of the large toe and the bottom of the large toe ball joint.

On the hands, the thymus reflex area is located along the medial edge about halfway between the wrist and the tip of the thumb, and is the same for both hands.

The thymus is responsible for making cells called *T-lymphocytes*, or *T-cells*, which have a big influence on our immune systems and overall strength. The lymphatic system carries white blood cells to the thymus, where they multiply and change into these special infection-fighting cells.

Although the function of the thymus is not fully understood, we know it plays an important part in developing immunities against various diseases. Many researchers believe the thymus produces the original lymphocytes formed in the body before birth and continues to produce them thereafter. The lymphocytes then travel from the thymus to the lymph nodes and spleen by way of the circulatory system. This shows how these organs all work together to form your immune system.

My first reflexology teacher and healing woman, Isabelle Hutton, told me to tap my thymus 100 times with my fingertips daily. She believes tapping the thymus stimulates it to produce more T-cells and, therefore, boost the immune system. If this is true, maybe this is why a hug feels so good. When we hug someone, we embrace the upper chest area, which is where the thymus sits.

### Foot Note

When we're born, our immune systems are not fully developed. Actually, our immune systems are not fully developed until about age 12. This is probably why children experience so many illnesses. I believe these early illnesses are nature's way of building up or exercising our immune system, if you will. Maybe that's why our thymus is larger when we're small, because it's working hard to build our immunity. After puberty, the thymus gland begins to shrink.

I tap my thymus every time I think about it, and I also try to get in as many daily hugs from my husband as I can. I figure even if it's a bunch of bologna, it still feels good and can't hurt a thing! So go give a hug to someone you love, and stimulate your immune system at the same time!

## The Least You Need to Know

◆ The main components of the immune system are the spleen, lymph system, and thymus.

◆ The liver compensates for a missing spleen, so it may be necessary to work on the liver reflex area of a person who has had their spleen removed.

◆ The immune system can be stimulated by tapping the thymus or giving hugs to the ones we love.

# 9

# A Lot to Swallow: The Digestive and Intestinal System

## In This Chapter

- ◆ Discover the importance of assimilation and elimination
- ◆ Learn to locate the reflex points for the digestive and intestinal organs
- ◆ Get to know the stomach, liver, gallbladder, and pancreas, and learn about some emotional links to your organs
- ◆ Meet your intestines
- ◆ Learn how to support your digestive health and feel better

Look through your medicine cabinet at home. What do you see? Over-the-counter medications for diarrhea, acid indigestion, heartburn, gas, constipation, and hemorrhoids? Well, well, well, these are all ailments of the intestinal and digestive tract, and the good news is that all these symptoms can be helped by using reflexology! Let's take a look at how these systems work together so you can get to working on yourself.

# Beginnings and Endings

How do you know when your intestinal and digestive systems are not working properly? Here are some clues:

- Heartburn, bloating, and belching

- Sour stomach and bad breath

- Intestinal gas

- Ulcers

- Always feeling hungry

- Constipation or diarrhea

- Appendicitis

- Being overweight or being severely underweight

- Acne, *rosacea*, or rashes

**def•i•ni•tion**

**Rosacea** is a skin disease in which the blood vessels in the cheeks and nose enlarge, causing the face to appear bright red or flushed. The cause is uncertain, but it's believed that extremes in temperature, food irritants, and too much alcohol can all play a part in aggravating the condition.

There's an old natural health saying: "Death begins in the colon." This is probably true. Our bowels are responsible for ridding us of harmful, toxic byproducts of digestion. It's the sewer system of the body. When the sewer system of a city is backed up, a health emergency is declared. When your body's sewer system is clogged up, your body also declares a health hazard—but you might not know how to interpret the signals.

This chapter helps you understand the importance of digesting, assimilating, and eliminating effectively. I discuss all the major organs of this system, including the stomach, liver, gallbladder, pancreas, and intestines. It's my favorite subject, and I hope you digest and absorb the information with ease.

# Where It All Starts: The Stomach

Although the first part of digestion starts when you begin chewing your food, I'm going to skip right down to talking about the stomach, where lots of churning goes on to digest the foods we eat.

The stomach is responsible for receiving food that's been partially digested by our saliva and chewing process. The stomach has already begun dumping digestive juices to prepare for the food coming down the tube. When the food arrives, the stomach walls actually mash, knead, and mix the food we eat with its digestive juices and prepare the mixture to be taken to its next stop—the small intestine. To break down proteins in foods, your stomach produces hydrochloric acid (HCl). Having a healthy amount of stomach acid is critical to keeping a strong digestive system and healthy body.

### Tip Toe

Hydrochloric acid supplements can help neutralize germs contained in our food and prevent stomach illness. Peppermint helps stimulate digestive juices and, therefore, aids digestion and may even help an upset stomach. I usually carry a small bottle of peppermint oil with me and put a dab on my tongue after meals. This not only helps my digestion but freshens my breath, too.

The stomach is located high up in your abdomen about in the middle of your left side, slightly extending into the right side of your body. It's somewhat protected by the left side of the rib cage. Each foot has a stomach reflex area, but it's primarily felt on the left foot (makes sense, doesn't it, as the stomach's primarily on the left side of the body?).

On the left foot, the stomach reflex area is found beginning just above the midline, or waist line, section of the foot, and extends inward toward the middle of the foot about halfway across. On the right foot, it's located in the same area but does not extend as far inward across the foot.

On the hands, the stomach area is predominately found on the left hand under the pointer finger, about halfway between the thumb and pointer finger, and extends a little more than halfway across the palm. On the right hand you can find it in the same area, but it does not extend as far across the palm.

> **Tip Toe**
>
> Does a person worry because of stomach problems, or does he get stomach problems because he worries too much? Either way, there's some evidence that the two are related. If you're experiencing troubles with your stomach, get some reflexology, and try not to worry about it. Your stomach will thank you.

In the following two figures, I've mapped out the entire digestive and intestinal system on the feet and hands so you can see the location of each reflex point.

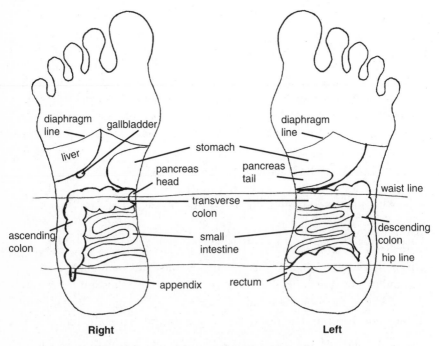

*The foot reflex points for the digestive and intestinal system.*

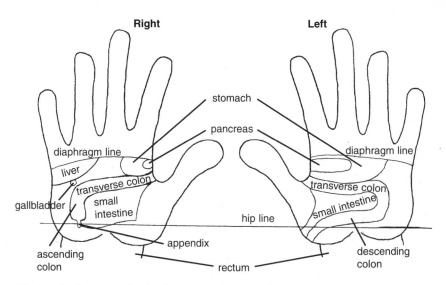

*The hand reflex points for the digestive and intestinal system.*

# Does Liver Live Here?

The digestive system relies on your liver to manufacture bile to digest fats, prevent constipation, and store sugar for future use. Your liver is located on the right side of your body, just under your diaphragm. The reflex area for the liver is located on the sole of your right foot beginning just about at the waist line area and extends from the outer ridge of your foot and across the foot to about the middle.

On the hands, the liver reflex area is located on the palm of your right hand just under the pad of the pinky finger and also extends across the palm toward the middle. There's also a reflex location on the top of your hand located at the point between the webbing of the thumb and first finger joint.

The liver has many functions, so it's appropriate that it's your largest organ, weighing an average of 3 pounds. It's a large, triangular, dark-colored organ that serves as a filter for all toxins (anything that isn't a natural substance) that enter your bloodstream. Some of the most common toxins include the following:

- Over-the-counter drugs
- Prescription medications
- Alcohol
- Food additives
- Chemicals
- Pesticides
- Preservatives

We expose our bodies to these substances every day and expect the liver to take care of us. But this filtering system is only one of its many functions. The liver reminds me of a faithful, hardworking employee who labors behind the scenes of a successful corporation. Like the valuable employee, the liver is often not acknowledged when it's doing its job, making sure the accounts are in order and everything is functioning smoothly. But when the worker gets worn out and starts letting things fall through the cracks, the rest of the system suffers, and the worker is blamed for his lack of efficiency!

If you work deeply on your liver reflex area and you feel a dull ache or pain in the reflex area, it could indicate that you have a sluggish liver. If your liver is overactive, on the other hand, you might feel more of a sharp pain when working on the liver reflex location. Working on this reflex helps your liver rebalance. If you experience either of these sensations when performing reflexology on the liver reflex area, it's a good idea to take a break from toxins for a few days.

Symptoms of an overburdened or stressed liver may include the following:

- Diarrhea
- Nausea
- Pimples
- Low-grade fever
- Mood swings
- Hepatitis
- Gallbladder trouble

Symptoms of an underactive or sluggish liver may include the following:

- Age spots
- Trouble falling asleep at night and waking up feeling unrested
- Anemia
- Bruising easily

- Body aches

- Mood swings

- Constipation

- Feeling cold and tired

- Poor digestion

- Food intolerance

- Sensitivity to strong odors

- Jaundice

**Tip Toe**

We can hold repressed anger energy in our liver, which is why when we cleanse the liver of its toxins, the release can have a toxic effect on our emotions! The middle finger is associated with the liver and gallbladder and is also the finger of anger. Coincidence?

The liver is not only our great filter, but it also serves to lubricate the intestines with bile. It's important for forming blood cells, producing hormones, and storing and utilizing vitamins and minerals.

# You Have Some Gallbladder

The gallbladder is a pear-shaped, greenish-looking organ located on the undersurface of the right lobe of the liver. The liver and gallbladder functions are intimately linked, as demonstrated by their close proximity to one another.

The gallbladder reflex location on the foot is just about in the middle of the liver reflex area, directly below the fourth toe, midway between the waist line and the diaphragm reflex line on the right foot. The right hand also contains the gallbladder point. This point is found directly below the fourth finger, about in the middle of the liver reflex area.

Basically, the gallbladder is just what its name says: a receptacle, or "bladder," that holds "gall," or bile. The gallbladder stores the gall and releases it through the bile duct to the upper part of the small intestine to aid in the breakdown of fats and oils. Our liver produces bile in response to fatty foods because bile emulsifies and breaks down these fats.

Loading up your diet with fat and greasy foods can cause the gallbladder to get behind in its work. Having to deal with so much grease can sometimes lead to the formation of *gallstones* or even a gallbladder attack! Some people I've known who have had gallbladder problems are convinced that reducing their fatty food intake would have been much less

**def•i•ni•tion**

A **gallstone** is a hard, stone-like mass made up of cholesterol (blood fat), bile pigments, and calcium salts. Gallstones can cause trouble when and if they get stuck in a bile duct, where they can cause jaundice.

painful than dealing with a gallbladder attack and consequent surgery.

If you're feeling wishy-washy and aren't able to make clear decisions on what you want to do in life, where you want to go, or how to get there, you could be experiencing sluggish gallbladder energy.

Working on the gallbladder area not only stimulates its function and balance in the body, but also helps us take charge and have the courage to understand that we must take responsibility for ourselves to make our lives what we want them to be.

# The Pancreas: Your Sweet-Tooth Organ

The pancreas is another organ that serves many functions. This pinkish, semi-oblong organ about 6 to 8 inches in length is located on the left side of your body midway between your diaphragm and your waist, a little behind and below your stomach.

The reflex point for the pancreas is located on the sole of each foot, but the area is larger on the left foot. It's located just under the stomach reflex point on the left foot and runs from the inside of the foot just about halfway across to the center of the foot, stopping at about the third toe. On the right foot, the spot is the same, but it doesn't run across as far as the left foot point, and it stops under the big toe.

There are two areas of the pancreas, called the head and tail or the head and body. The pancreas head and body serve different primary functions. The head of the pancreas mainly serves our digestion and is responsible for making enzymes to help us break down our foods. These enzymes break down starches, fats, and proteins and change them to sugars and amino acids. The tail or body of the pancreas is most active in making insulin. Insulin is produced to keep our blood sugar levels adequate and regulated.

Because the pancreas helps us regulate our blood sugar levels, it's an important part of the digestive system. Pancreatic fluid neutralizes HCl and protects us from getting ulcers. The pancreas also has a hand in manufacturing hormones and regulating blood sugar.

When the pancreas is not up to par, our blood sugar level can rise dangerously high and can even lead to brain damage and death. High blood sugar, or *hyperglycemia*, that becomes chronic is known as *diabetes*. When the pancreas is overproducing insulin, the blood sugar level can become too low and the result is *hypoglycemia*. Lack of blood sugar is just as dangerous as high blood sugar, because the brain uses blood sugar, also known as *glucose*, as its constant food supply.

---

**Tip Toe**

Emotionally, the pancreas is related to our childlike qualities and to the sweetness of life and how we experience it. When the pancreas points are stimulated on the feet, it not only helps the body digest better and balance blood sugar levels, but it may also help us get back in touch with the child in us who needs to come out and play!

---

# Where It All Ends: The Colon

The intestinal system includes the small and large intestines (the colon), which serve similar functions and are part of the same food tube that started back at the stomach. The small intestine is a tubelike organ that's been described as an elaborate food processor. It forms a winding mass located in your trunk cavity between your waist and hips. The primary function of the small intestine is the digestion and assimilation of nutrients, and this is where most of the nutrients from the food and supplements we eat are absorbed.

The small intestine reflex area spans the width of the entire foot from the waist line to the hip line area. (As you'll see, there are many overlapping areas on the feet and hands, just as our body organs are in overlapping areas.)

The colon, or large intestine, is also a tubelike organ, approximately 5 feet long, but wider in diameter than the small intestine. Its shape is not unlike an upside-down U. The primary function of the colon, or large intestine, is the elimination of solid waste materials. The reflex area for the large intestine is broken down into three distinct areas: the ascending colon, the transverse colon, and the descending colon (known as the sigmoid), ending at the rectum reflex location.

The ascending colon begins on the lower side of the right foot, just above the heel about midway between the fourth and fifth toes, going up to about mid-foot. It then takes a sharp turn toward the opposite foot and extends all the way across the foot to the instep. It picks up again on the left foot, reflecting the transverse colon starting at about the waist line. Then it spans across the foot to almost under the baby toe and down the descending colon, making one more turn just above the heel back out toward the instep to the rectum reflex area.

Not surprisingly, the lower colon is where I seem to find most of the "crunchies" in people's feet. The most common area of congestion in the colon may be the area where the descending colon makes its final turn before heading to the rectum (the sigmoid).

Wastes tend to accumulate at the bottom of the descending colon, and this reflex area, on the left foot just below the hip line, is tender for most people. Many of us are constipated without even knowing it. The colon has an amazing ability to hold on to waste materials and harbor poisons. Like the stomach, the colon can expand as more waste backs up into it. Portions of the bowel can even push outward, making little bowel pockets. The fecal matter caught in these pockets can fester and inflame, causing a disease known as *diverticulitis*.

## def•i•ni•tion

**Diverticulitis** is a disease of the bowel where compacted fecal matter causes pressure in the bowel that produces small pouches, or bowel pockets, along the intestinal walls. These sacs can fester and inflame, causing severe discomfort. These infected pockets can be dangerous or deadly if they burst.

The role the colon plays in the body deserves a lot of attention and consideration in your health programs. The colon is your body's sewer system, and it's important to your health that you keep it moving. I've found that reflexology can be a fabulous therapy for stimulating the lower bowel into action. So those rumors about reflexologists emptying your pockets might just be true after all!

# Constipation: When Things Are *Not* Moving

It's not uncommon during reflexology treatments to hear the stomach and intestines begin to growl. The growling is actually a good sign, because it means you're moving energy. If shortly after beginning a treatment, strange noises begin to emerge from beneath the blanket, you can guess that the digestive track is being stimulated into action and the bowel is preparing for elimination.

I've had success with helping people overcome constipation and also spastic bowel conditions using reflexology. In addition, nausea has subsided during the administration of reflexology. A backup of bowel toxins causes some headaches; stimulating the bowel reflex points on the feet and hands can relieve those headaches by allowing the bowel to evacuate promptly.

Constipation can be relieved with reflexology by stimulating the following reflexes:

- ◆ Ascending colon
- ◆ Transverse colon
- ◆ Descending colon
- ◆ Small intestine
- ◆ Liver

Headaches or nausea caused by constipation require the same reflex stimulation with the addition of the brain, neck, and head areas.

Another frequent complaint that can be related to constipation is adult acne. More women than men seem to experience this annoying ailment. The first question that should come to mind when faced with this problem is "How often do you frequent the bathroom?"

If the answer is once per day or less, consider focusing on the bowel reflex points. The skin is as clean as the blood is, and the blood is as clean as the bowel. Therefore, cleansing the bowel should get at the root cause of the adult acne problem.

The best way to avoid diseases of the bowel is to keep your elimination channels clear. Getting reflexology treatments, drinking plenty of water, eating fibrous foods such as whole fruits and vegetables, taking herbal supplements, exercising, and listening to the call of nature in a timely manner all help keep your bowel functioning properly!

## The Least You Need to Know

◆ Improper functioning of the digestive system can rob your body of important nutrients and lead to an array of illnesses.

◆ Your stomach is central to the digestive process.

◆ Your liver helps break down fats and serves as the major filter in your body.

◆ Your pancreas regulates your blood sugar levels, and its fluid protects you from intestinal ulcers.

◆ Your colon is your body's sewer system and it must be kept clean for proper health.

◆ Reflexology, correct eating habits, and supplementation are all part of a preventative health program for your digestive and intestinal system.

# 10

# Down to the Bone: The Structural System

## In This Chapter

♦ Learn about the structural system

♦ Locate the structural reflex areas on the feet and hands

♦ Learn how reflexology can benefit your structural system

♦ Understand how reflexology can help jaw and tooth pain

> The body has three important bones: The wish bone, because everyone needs hopes, dreams, and goals; the funny bone, because everything in life has to be mixed with a dose of humor; and a back bone, to give people strength to stand up for what they believe in.
>
> —Words of wisdom taken from a Nampa, Idaho, Chamber of Commerce Newsletter

Can you imagine not having any bones? Just think, the old movie *The Blob* wouldn't make any sense to us. We would have to purchase our clothes from beanbag manufacturers. Instead of rocking, we'd just have to roll. And don't even think about the Jell-O and tofu jokes we'd have to endure!

# A Structured Environment

Our structural system is made up of more than just bones, but our bones give our body the structural framework on which to hang our flesh. The structural system actually encompasses the muscles, cartilage, joints, tendons, teeth, skin, and even the hair and nails. The bones give our body the ability to stand and perform intricate movements.

The body contains a total of 206 bones. If you remember from Chapter 3, the feet and hands contain more than half the bones in the entire body. In addition to keeping us upright, our bones serve as protectors, encasing our delicate organs and keeping them from being easily exposed to damage.

Many ailments are associated with structural system imbalance, including the following:

◆ Arthritis

◆ Rheumatoid arthritis

◆ Osteoarthritis

◆ Osteoporosis

◆ Bursitis

◆ Cracking and popping of joints

◆ Muscle cramps

◆ Back pain

◆ Brittle hair and/or fingernails

◆ Tooth decay

Several reflex points on the feet and hands correspond to the structural system. The main ones are the spine, including the neck, the joints (knee, hip, elbow, shoulder), and the jaw and teeth. I address each reflex area when we check out those particular joints, but for now you can look at the following foot and hand diagrams to see the main components of the structural system mapped out.

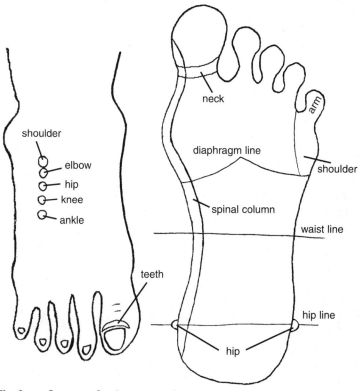

*The foot reflex areas for the structural system.*

*The hand reflex areas for the structural system.*

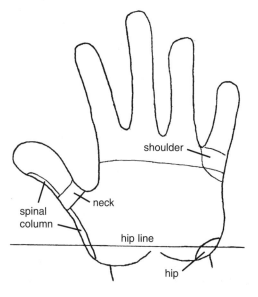

**Tip Toe**

Our bones and teeth are made up primarily of calcium. Skin, hair, and nails are made primarily of keratin and are nourished by silicon. Foods rich in both silicon and calcium include barley, beans, cauliflower, dandelion greens, millet, whole wheat, and onions.

# Having the Backbone to Get Treatment

The spine is literally and figuratively our backbone. We use it to stand upright and to take a stand, or a bow, as the case may be. The spine reflex can be found along the instep of each foot going all the way up to the top of the big toe, which is the head area. The neck area wraps around the entire base of the big toe. On each hand, the spine area can be found all along the outside edge of the thumb side of the hand (medial edge), running from the wrist on up to the top of the thumb.

## Foot Note

When my husband and I were in Mexico on a vacation, I woke up one morning with a terribly stiff neck. The pain severely restricted my movement. We were determined not to let this problem spoil our fun, so we headed to the white, sandy beach where my helpful husband worked on my neck reflexes on my big toes as I worked on my hand reflexes. These spots were very tender, and we concentrated only on the neck and spine areas for 1 hour. I began to feel improvement right away, and after the hour was up, the kink in my neck was relieved and we were able to go scuba diving that afternoon!

Reflexology treatments help relax the muscles along and around the spine and back area, which can help ease back pain. I was taught to massage the reflexes for the whole spine for at least 1 to 2 minutes, although it can be "reflexed" indefinitely. This helps improve the entire circulatory system and relieve muscle tension throughout the entire body. Relaxing the muscles also helps restore the proper functioning and alignment of the spinal column.

The spine, running from the tailbone up to the base of the neck to the skull, consists of 25 bones called *vertebrae*. The spine's vertebrae are held together by ligaments and intervertebral disks, making it a flexible structure. It's a complicated structure housing an intricate network of nerves. Technically, the spine is also part of the nervous system because it houses our inner wiring system of nerves.

Running through our spine is the *spinal cord*, literally the main cable to our central nervous system. All messages sent from the brain to the rest of the body filter through this amazing electrical network of nerves running through and along our spine. Therefore, the correct alignment of the spine is crucial for maintaining clear communication signals to the rest of the body.

# Need a Realignment?

Working the spine reflex area on the feet and hands is especially important because each vertebra also affects a different organ in the body through a reflex point. If a certain vertebra is out of alignment, meaning it is out of its normal place, the electrical impulses that run through that particular vertebra can be pinched off.

*Subluxation* (or the misalignment of a joint) may not only cause discomfort, but it can also mean that the reflex organ is not getting clear signals from the brain. Nor can the associated organ receive the adequate blood supply needed for nourishment and oxygen imperative for healthy function.

Why does a vertebra go out of alignment? Many times a muscle imbalance or spasm is the culprit. Just think of the multitudes of employees who work on computers these days, either at their work, as their work, or even for entertainment. Because of this, many of us suffer with what my computer consultant husband calls *mouse shoulder*. Mouse shoulder is when the shoulder muscles behind our shoulder blades spasm or tighten, creating a pull on the upper spine that pulls a vertebra out of its normal place.

**def•i•ni•tion**

**Subluxation** is the fancy word for any joint being out of alignment. If you visit a chiropractor, she or he will usually diagnose you with one or more subluxations along your spinal column. Reflexology can help chiropractic adjustments last longer by keeping the muscles relaxed. Don't be lax about spinal care!

When working on the spine, it's always helpful to find the cause of the problem and eliminate it first. Then help the body recover with natural therapies such as reflexology. Sometimes an old injury, such as whiplash, leaves a weakened area along your spine. Or damage to the ligaments could leave the vertebra vulnerable to misalignment in a particular area. Many things can cause this, including lifting something too heavy or making sudden, twisting movements like you would playing golf or softball.

Whether working on yourself or another, you're usually able to tell where the spine is out of alignment. When you're working on someone and you find a crunchy or a tender spot along the spine reflex area, this is a good indication of a subluxation. When I find a tender area on the foot, let's say on the lower spine area, I ask the client if their lower back is sore. They always answer with a surprised "Yes!" and some think I'm a fortune-teller! The analysis can be amazingly accurate. Try it on yourself and see.

# One Classy Joint

The joints in the body are the areas where two bones meet. The joints I cover here are the major ones, including the shoulder, elbow, hip, knee, and jaw, which is home to the *temporal mandibular joint*, better known as *TMJ*.

### def•i•ni•tion

The **temporal mandibular joint,** known commonly as **TMJ,** is the hinge joint where the mandibular bone (jaw) and the temporal bone (one of the skull bones) articulate together. Discuss TMJ problems, such as popping, clicking, or pain, with your dentist for guidance.

Our joints offer us flexibility and help us move in an array of amazing positions. We already visualized not having bones, but what if we didn't have joints? We would all move like Barbie and Ken dolls. How would we get our socks off to get a reflexology treatment?

The reflex points that correspond to the joints are located on the top of the foot, between the anklebone and the fourth and fifth toes. Closest to the toes is the ankle reflex. Next are the knee, hip, elbow, and shoulder.

These areas are all part of a rectangular area that encompasses all the joints for that particular side of the body. Technically, these areas are not reflex points, but I want to break them down so I can talk a little bit about each. If you work this general area all along the points you see on the diagram earlier in the chapter, you will positively affect all your joints.

Let's talk a little more about them individually.

## Lay Your Thumb on My Shoulder

Your shoulders are ball socket joints, meaning that one end of the bone is round like a ball, which fits snugly into a divot, or socket-shaped bone. Ball joints offer more flexibility than hinge joints, which can only move back and forth in one direction. The ball joint in the shoulder offers your arms a great range of movement.

On the sole of the foot, the shoulder joint reflex is located all along the base of the little toe and down toward the diaphragm line. The little toe symbolizes the arm. On the hand, the shoulder reflex area is located all along the base of the pinky finger and down toward the diaphragm line. The pinky symbolizes the arm, and the rest of the fingers represent themselves.

The shoulder gives you flexibility. My mouse shoulder always responds positively when I rub deeply on the shoulder reflex area on my hand. My husband works on the shoulder reflex area on my feet, which is always crunchy! After he's done digging his thumb into my shoulder reflex point, I thank him because my neck and shoulders feel better immediately.

This is what I generally find with reflexology. When the discomfort in the reflex area subsides, so does the discomfort in the corresponding body part.

## Reflexology Is a Hip Therapy

Your hip joints are the region of the body where the leg bones connect to your pelvis. The hipbones are located on either side of your ... well ... hips! The hip line on the reflex charts in this book gives you a reference point across the heel, but the actual hip reflexes are located all around the outer ankle bones and on each side of the heel.

I also think it benefits my clients when I work from one side of the heel all along the hip reflex line. This helps relieve lower back and pelvis pain and releases tension in the hips. The hip reflexes in the hands are located around the wrist bone on the "pinky" side of each wrist.

Here's a hip tip to see how much tension you're holding in your hips: when you lay down on your back and relax, see which way your feet fall. Do they stay basically straight up and down, or do they fall inward or in opposite directions? You can suspect tension in the hips when both feet fall to the outside. This usually means the muscles in the outer thighs and hips are tightened and are effectively pulling the feet outward. Working on the hip reflex area over a period of time should change this tension and bring the feet back to the middle.

## A Knee-Jerk Reaction

The knee joint is formed by the lower end of the *femur* (the large leg bone) and the upper ends of the *tibia* and *fibula* (the shin bones), and also includes the *patella* (kneecap). Your knees are subjected to a tremendous amount of lateral stress during normal activity throughout your life. The knee is guarded by a number of ligaments to lend it support.

**def•i•ni•tion**

The **femur, tibia** and **fibula,** and **patella** are all bones of the leg. The patella is the kneecap, the femur is the largest leg bone, and the tibia and fibula make up the shins.

Many of us participate in sporting activities such as jogging, skiing, and gymnastics, which can put much more stress on our knees than they're able to handle. Therefore, lots of us have knee problems at one time or another. Reflex areas for the knee joints are located on top of the foot about midway between the anklebone and the webbing of the fourth and fifth toes.

The reflex for the knees is midway between the wrist and the fourth and fifth knuckles on the top (dorsal) side of each hand (not shown in the figures earlier in this chapter). Pinching the outside (pinky side) area of each hand works the lateral sides of the body and helps loosen excess tension in the knees.

The knee reflexes on the feet are also located on the dorsal (top) side of each foot between the ankle and the fourth and fifth toes. When the knee joints are having trouble, a gentle massage directly around the knee may prove beneficial. Usually reflexology stimulates better circulation to the knees, which helps the knees heal.

## Go Ahead, Twist My Arm

Without the elbow, we'd all be in straight-armed trouble and have to really think about how we'd get food into our mouths, brush our teeth, scratch our noses, etc. With all that bending and twisting, it's easy to see why the elbow needs a little rest and reflexology work sometimes.

The elbow reflex point on the foot is located on the top part of the foot about midway between the anklebone and the webbing between the fourth and fifth toes (closer to the toes). Another area that covers the elbow is the little toe, which corresponds to the entire arm. The left baby toe corresponds to the left arm, and the right to the right. Similarly, the elbow reflex point on the hands is found on each pinky finger, which corresponds to the whole arm.

## Muscling In

As I mentioned earlier, the structural system is not just made of bones, but also muscles and tendons that give you the power to move your bones. Your muscles rely on magnesium and a balance of other minerals to keep them healthy.

Your muscles also like to be stretched slowly. This helps them take in a healthy blood supply and keep the circulation going so you don't get stiff and achy. Reflexology helps relax all your muscles and helps increase the circulation to your whole body, which is another reason it makes you feel so good.

# The Whole Tooth

Of course your teeth aren't joints, but they do fall under the umbrella of the structural system. The bones that support your teeth come together at the side of your face just under your ears and make up the joint known as TMJ (temporal mandibular joint).

Clicking and popping of the temporal mandibular joint can indicate TMJ problems, which can be caused by clenching or grinding your teeth. Many times stress and worry cause you to grind or clench your teeth, especially at night. (In this case, a night-guard made for you by your dentist might be helpful to prevent damage to your teeth and jaw while you deal with the source of your stress.) There can be other causes as well. Sometimes a filling can be too high, for example, and cause your jaw to close crookedly, which can lead to painful jaw and TMJ problems.

Reflexology can help with TMJ problems by relaxing the muscles associated with the clenching. Your teeth exert a tremendous pressure when you grind or clench them. This can damage the structure of your teeth and even trigger migraines and other headaches.

> **Tip Toe**
>
> Many people hold their thumbs when getting their teeth worked on. If you hold tightly on to the teeth reflexes on your thumbs the next time you're at your dentist, you can help stop discomfort. Some people have gone as far as wearing rubberbands around the base of their thumbnails to alleviate dental discomfort.

The jaw and teeth reflex areas are located on top of the big toe on each foot. The teeth and jaw points run along the area just below the base of the big toenail and up slightly on each side. The jaw and teeth reflex points on the hand run just below the base of the thumbnail on both hands.

The thumb is also associated with worry. I think babies suck their thumbs because it pacifies them. Pressing tightly on the tooth and jaw reflex areas on the thumbs just might serve to pacify any nervousness you might feel, too. Later I get into specific techniques, but for now, hold on to those thumbs.

## The Least You Need to Know

♦ The structural system supports the entire body and is made up of bones, cartilage, tendons, ligaments, and muscles.

◆ The alignment of your spine affects blood supply and electrical impulse distribution to the rest of your organs. Reflexology can help prolong your chiropractic spinal adjustments by relaxing your back muscles.

◆ The joints are where the bones come together, and, along with our muscles and tendons, allow us to bend, twist, and move easily. Reflexology can restore circulation to the joints, which can aid healing.

◆ Stretching after a reflexology treatment enhances the therapeutic effects of the treatment by helping maintain flexibility and aiding the muscles to release toxins by bringing in a fresh blood supply.

◆ Reflex points below the base of the thumb correspond to the teeth and jaw and can be used to ease the discomfort of TMJ problems and help calm nerves when visiting the dentist.

# What Nerve!: The Nervous System

## In This Chapter

- ◆ Learn about your brain
- ◆ Locate the nervous system reflexes on your feet and hands
- ◆ Get to know your pituitary and pineal glands
- ◆ Understand how your adrenals affect your energy levels and how stress affects your adrenals
- ◆ Benefit from the calming effects of reflexology

Technically, the components of the nervous system consist of the brain and spinal column. I talked about the spine as part of the structural system in Chapter 10, so throughout the text and in this chapter, I "borrowed" some glands from the endocrine system and sprinkled them in with other systems where appropriate. Stress, nervousness, and tension all are connected with the hormones that the adrenals produce, so I discuss them here under the nervous system. And the pineal and pituitary are glands, but they're located *in* the brain, so I discuss them here as well. If you take a reflexology class, however, you will most likely be taught about the adrenals and the pituitary and pineal glands as part of the endocrine system.

Imbalances in the nervous system (including problems with the pituitary and/or pineal glands) can go to either end of the emotional scale, meaning that disturbances can be felt as highs, known as *mania*, or lows in the form of *depression*. Nervous system imbalances may include the following:

- Anxiety
- Depression
- Memory loss
- Alzheimer's disease
- ADD (attention deficit disorder)
- Speech pattern disturbances
- Mental illness
- Premature aging

Any or all these ailments may be linked to nervous system malfunctions due to malnutrition, something in the present or past environment, or chemical imbalances due to glandular malfunction. Here I discuss working the reflexes that help stimulate your body to balance, which can be of benefit for all these ailments.

# The Brain: Thinking on Your Feet

Studying the brain must be similar to being on the road to knowledge and enlightenment: the more you learn, the more you realize that there's a lot you don't know. Scientists, psychologists, and neuroscientists studying the brain make new discoveries and uncover more amazing facts about how the brain actually works, which leads to further experimentation.

# King Brain

The brain is the primary component of the nervous system. It's connected to the upper end of the spinal cord and is responsible for issuing nerve impulses, processing nerve impulse data, and engaging in the higher-order thought processes.

Positioned at the top of the body, literally and figuratively, the brain is the king of the hill. And it works hard for its position. The brain serves more functions than we might ever be able to discover. Along with the heart, the brain is the organ most vital for sustaining life.

The brain uses more nutrients, oxygen, and glucose (blood sugar) than any other organ, and it also has first dibs on these nutrients. In the internal world, the brain is the king, and the blood carries the oxygen and nutrients to it first. When the king is done feasting, the blood redistributes the nutrients to the other organs in the body.

---

### Foot Note

The brain and the mind are different things. The brain is our computer, and scientists are finding out exactly how it functions. However, the mind remains a mystery. Although we know how impulses are sent to different parts of our body when we have a thought, we really don't know where the original thought is generated. Who or what is really doing the thinking? Where does inspiration come from? These are the secrets of the mind that continue to give us thoughts to ponder.

---

The reflex points for the brain are located at the very tips of the toes. The large toe especially reflects the brain, because the large toe represents the head. The same goes for the brain reflex area on the hands, located at the tip of each finger and especially the top of the thumb.

The following figures show the reflex points for the brain area along with some other glands that affect the nervous system.

# Treat Your Brain Well

You can be good to your brain in many different ways. Physical exercise helps bring more oxygen to the blood, a vital nutrient needed for clear thinking and alertness. When you're lacking oxygen in the blood, the brain's functions are not as sharp. You get lethargic, and you might feel mentally slow-moving, too. Reflexology helps by increasing the circulation to the brain so it can receive the oxygen and nutrients it needs.

*The foot reflex points that affect the nervous system, along with two glands located in the brain: the pineal and pituitary. These same reflexes are located on both feet.*

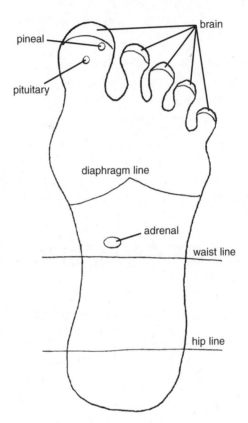

*The hand reflex points that affect the nervous system. These same reflexes are found on both hands.*

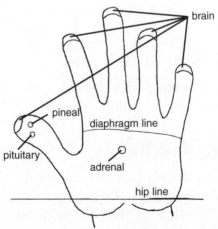

Without adequate stimulation, the brain can become sluggish and actually start to calcify. This calcification literally hardens parts of our brains and can make us stubborn, set in our ways, and extremely inflexible.

The good news is that studies indicate that with proper stimulation, our brains can continue to grow and we can increase our intelligence and brain function well into our 70s, 80s, and 90s! Regular reflexology treatments, along with exercise, mental challenges, proper nutrients, and positive thoughts, keep us in a positive frame of mind and keep our brains and our bodies feeling younger and more alive.

**Tip Toe**

Adequate rest is an important part of recharging not only your mind, but the rest of your body. Although the brain never sleeps, your conscious mind requires time off nightly to keep you alert and functioning during the daytime.

# The Pituitary: Master Controller

The pituitary gland is a small, pea-size ball of tissue hanging from a tiny, stemlike piece of flesh from the underside of the brain. Because of its location in the brain, I have categorized the pituitary under the nervous system in this book. However, this tiny gland is actually part of the endocrine system or *glandular system*. The pituitary affects myriad functions, and the messages it sends control all other glandular functions. You might consider the pituitary a little guy with a big control issue!

**def•i•ni•tion**

The **glandular system** is a general term used to describe all the glands of the body. The glandular system is divided into two categories: the endocrine glands (without ducts) and the exocrine glands (with ducts). Glands are organs or groups of cells that make and secrete fluids, such as hormones.

The pituitary helps send messages to the rest of the glandular system and regulates growth mechanisms, skin pigmentation, blood pressure, and sexual development. This gland is also responsible for the prevention of an excessive accumulation of fat.

Imbalances of the pituitary gland can manifest in a variety of ways, including the following:

◆ Obesity

◆ Growth problems

◆ Hindered or excessive body development

◆ Sexual development disturbances

◆ High or low blood pressure

◆ Feelings of moroseness or depression

The reflex for the pituitary gland can be found on each large toe. To locate it, find the bull's-eye of the swirl in your big toe print. To stimulate this gland, push up and then in toward the center of the toe at the same time.

You'll know when you stimulate this point because you'll feel either an electric shock or like someone has stuck a pin into your toe. This sharp reaction is especially noticeable in people who have calcium deposits building up in their brain.

As for the hands, the pituitary gland reflex is found on each thumb. To locate it, use the same method as for the toe: find the middle of the swirl on the thumbprint, and push up and in toward the middle of the thumb to stimulate it.

Feeling ill-humored and depressed? That can be caused by an improperly functioning pituitary gland. Stimulating this gland with reflexology just might be the key to alleviating depression and lifting your spirits!

---

### Foot Note

*Glandular body typing* is a method for analyzing a person based on his or her particular glandular body type. Invented by Dr. Henry Bieler, M.D., and expanded on by the Tree of Light Institute in Utah, this method identifies the dominant gland in your body—identified by your body shape and general characteristics. For instance, a pituitary type tends to have most of his energy in his head, tending to be intellectual and idealistic. The pituitary type looks young for her age, has smallish features, and is shorter in stature. Usually these people have rounded shoulders, beautiful teeth, get baby fat all over when overweight, and women tend to be small-breasted.

# The Pineal: Seeing the Light of Day

One of the least-understood glands in the body is the pineal. This gland is also part of the endocrine or glandular system, but it's located in the brain so I'm talking about it here.

The pineal is located just behind and slightly above the pituitary gland. The reflex point for the pineal is located on the upper quadrant of each big toe. In relation to the pituitary gland reflex, the pineal gland reflex is a little bit closer to the second toe and slightly above the pituitary reflex point. The stimulation of this reflex is also felt as a sharp zing, but this feeling is usually duller than the zing of the pituitary reflex point.

> **Foot Note**
>
> The pineal gland can calcify. Usually this is found in old age if it happens at all. Calcification of this gland has been linked to the slowing down and aging of the rest of the body and to a general deterioration in health.

On the hand, the pineal reflex point can be found on each thumb, slightly toward the pointer finger from the pituitary reflex point. (See the figure earlier in this chapter to find the general location.) These spots are both hard to locate when you work on yourself, but after you hit them, the "zing" lets you know you've found them!

Your pineal gland is a bit of a mystery. Many believe it's responsible for dreams and even psychic abilities. We do know that it's responsible for producing and regulating the hormone *melatonin* in the body. This hormone has been linked to *seasonal affective disorder*, or *SAD*, a syndrome characterized by severe depression brought on by a lack of sunshine. Many suffer from this disorder in areas where it tends to be overcast or dark during the winter months.

## def•i•ni•tion

> **Seasonal affective disorder,** otherwise known as **SAD,** is a syndrome characterized by severe depression during certain times of the year. Most notably, the depression is experienced during times when there is a lack of sunshine. This disorder brings on a desire to overeat, especially refined carbohydrates which can stimulate serotonin release in the brain. Stimulating the pineal gland may help SAD people.

Melatonin also regulates our sleep patterns, making us feel sleepy when nighttime comes. Ideally, sunlight *should* suppress the brain's production of melatonin so we feel fresh and alert each morning, but we know this isn't always the case!

When you feel the "blahs" coming on, especially on dark or overcast days, give your pineal reflex point a few good zings and see if it doesn't help clear your mental fog.

# Adrenals: Fight or Flight

The adrenals, located atop your kidneys, are also glands, making them part of the glandular system—but again, I discuss them here under the nervous system because they produce chemicals that affect the nervous system and are greatly affected by stress. They are very small glands, only about as large as the tip of your pinky finger and weighing about as much as a coin.

The adrenals have an influence on your vigor, sense of courage, vitality, and fervor. They are linked to your ability to work hard, get excited, and even stick up for yourself and influence the immune, digestive, hormonal, mineral, and entire glandular balance. However, physical and mental stresses can lead to the weakening of the adrenals, as can the overuse of caffeine and other stimulants.

> ### Tread Lightly
> If you find an indented adrenal reflex point, you might suspect a digestive problem. Reflexology isn't meant to diagnose, but you might want to consider digestive disturbances or gallbladder or liver ailments that sometimes indicate a metabolizing imbalance. You should also check the gallbladder and liver reflex areas for tenderness for more clues. Also, if the adrenals are weak, most likely the thyroid will be affected as well.

The adrenals produce a hormone called, appropriately, *adrenaline*—your flight or fight response hormone. When you're under a great deal of stress, or whatever you perceive to be a great deal of stress, the adrenals pump out adrenaline and *noradrenaline*, which have an immediate and profound effect on your body, preparing you for a fight or for flight—running from danger. Too much stress keeps the adrenals on constant call, which can eventually weaken them and make you feel lethargic and even depressed.

The adrenal reflex points are located on the soles of both feet, about mid-foot, slightly above the waist line area. The adrenal reflex points on the hand are located slightly above the midpoint of the palm. So if, in the middle of a stressful day, you find yourself wanting energy and looking for a candy bar or other stimulant for a boost, you might try stimulating your adrenal reflex points first. It's a healthier alternative to caffeine or a sugary snack.

## The Least You Need to Know

♦ The pineal gland is located in the brain and is associated with our sleep/wake cycles, dreaming, and even aging. Proper functioning of this gland may keep you young.

♦ The adrenal glands regulate your fight or flight response when you experience stress. Using reflexology may help reduce fatigue brought on by weak adrenals.

♦ Because of its overall affect on the glandular and nervous systems, reflexology is a great therapy for anxiety and depression and may aid in balancing out the highs and lows that come from high-stress lives.

# Chapter 12

# Remember to Breathe: The Respiratory System

## In This Chapter

- Discover the functions of the respiratory system
- Learn how emotions may be linked to respiratory illness
- Locate the respiratory system reflexes on the feet and hands
- Breathe better with reflexology
- Help your eyes and ears: improve the respiratory system

Take a long, slow, deep breath and then exhale. Did your shoulders rise when you inhaled? Did you have to open your mouth to get in enough air to take that deep breath? Or did you have to exhale first? Most of us could improve our respiratory function by freeing ourselves of tension, allergies, asthma, or other respiratory problems. When we don't breathe as well as we should, we can become lethargic. Let's take a look at how reflexology can ease some of these problems and get you breathing deep and feeling better!

# Divine Respiration

The primary functions of the respiratory system include breathing, filtering dust particles, warming the body, humidifying, and exchanging oxygen with carbon dioxide. Starting from the nose, the major organs of the respiratory system I cover in this chapter consist of the sinus cavities, bronchi, lungs, and diaphragm.

In this chapter, I also talk about the eyes and ears. Although these are sensory organs, they're situated very close to the sinus cavities. When we have a respiratory ailment—such as allergies, for instance—the eyes itch and water and the ears feel plugged because of this proximity. I find that working the eye and ear reflex points helps my clients greatly when they have allergy-related symptoms.

When the respiratory system is not up to par, energy lags. The respiratory system also serves as a line of defense, protecting the body from harmful airborne toxins. It also serves as an elimination channel, carrying out waste products.

Ailments of the respiratory system include the following:

◆ Sinusitis

◆ Allergies

◆ Asthma

◆ Bronchitis

◆ Pneumonia

◆ Emphysema

Now take a deep breath as we dive into the major components of the respiratory system.

# A Little Heavy Breathing: The Lungs

The lungs are located in the chest cavity on the left and right sides of the body and are protected mostly by the rib cage. The *bronchi* are the airways to each lung and are divided into even smaller airways called *bronchioles*. The exchange of oxygen into carbon dioxide takes place in the *alveoli* (air pockets) in the terminal ends of the bronchioles.

## def•i•ni•tion

The **bronchi** are the airways to the lungs and are divided into even smaller airways called **bronchioles**. The bronchioles allow the exchange of air and waste gases between the alveoli and the bronchi. **Alveoli** are small pockets that stick out along the walls of alveolar sacs in the lungs. This is where carbon dioxide leaves the blood and the blood takes in oxygen.

The reflex areas for the lungs and bronchi cover almost the entire ball of the foot (the padding under the toes) and also the space between the metatarsal bones on the top and bottom of each foot. This entire area on both feet represents the chest area of the body. The bronchial tube reflexes run from the ball of the foot just under the inside edge of each large toe and up to the base of the large toe on each foot.

On the hands, the lung area covers about the whole area of the top part of the palm. Squeezing in between the webbing of the fingers on each hand also works the chest and lung and bronchi areas.

See the following hand and foot illustrations to see the respiratory system mapped out, along with the eyes and ears. Notice how many of these areas overlap.

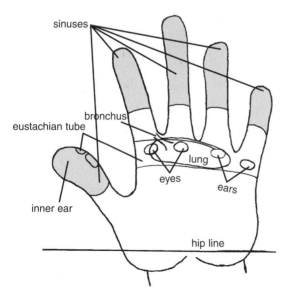

*The hand reflexes for the respiratory system, eyes, and ears. Reflexes are the same for both hands.*

*The foot reflexes for the respiratory system, eyes, and ears. Reflexes are the same for both feet.*

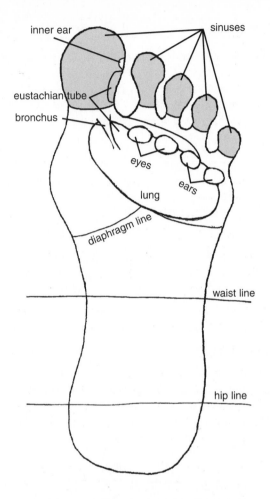

The reflexes in the left hand and foot are associated with the left lung, eye, ear, bronchi, and sinuses. The reflexes on the right hand and foot correlate to the organs on the right side of the body.

## Eliminate the Negative

In addition to supplying essential oxygen to the body, the lungs carry out gaseous wastes such as carbon dioxide and cellular byproducts, which make them one of our elimination channels. The lungs can also expel tiny irritants, such as dust particles or fungi. The respiratory system coats these particles with mucus and then evicts them through coughing.

**Tip Toe**

Chinese ephedra (Ma Haung) is a controversial herb used for centuries to help asthmatics breathe. It's an ingredient used in many herbal combinations designed to aid the respiratory system. Ephedra is a heart and nervous system stimulant and is not suitable for everyone, which is why it's been banned in some states. Please ask your physician before using this herb.

Despite all this important activity, the lungs actually are passive, meaning they do not move on their own. The diaphragm, the muscle below the lungs just under the ribs, moves up and down, pushing air out of the lungs and allowing the lungs to fill back up. The diaphragm reflex lies just below the ball of each foot. The reference line shown as the diaphragm line in this book's figures is the actual diaphragm reflex area. You work this area by following the line all the way across the base of the ball of the foot with your thumb. (See Chapter 5 to learn how to use finger and thumb techniques.)

On each hand, the diaphragm reference line is also the same as the actual diaphragm reflex area. It spans the bottom of the padding of each hand. When you're short of breath or tense, this whole area on the feet and hands will usually be tender and feel tense. Rub these areas until your body and lungs relax, especially if you're short of breath from nervous tension.

When the lungs aren't eliminating properly, where do you think the gaseous wastes and particles go? Some continue circulating in the bloodstream, keeping your immune system working overtime and leaving you even more vulnerable to illness. Some of these waste products settle back into the tissues of the body. Settled toxins can later cause irritations, such as allergies or what seems to be a cold, to affect your respiratory channels.

**Foot Note**

Deep-breathing exercises can increase your capacity to eliminate old toxins from your body. These exercises are helpful to do during a reflexology treatment, especially when you're working on the lung areas. After the treatment, breathing deeply assists the elimination process for the lungs and upper respiratory system and aids the whole body in its elimination and uptake of oxygen.

## Good Grief, It's Asthma

Emotionally speaking, the lungs are associated with grief. Many times, folks with chronic allergies or asthma who haven't gotten well in response to reflexology and other forms of treatment are holding on to unexpressed sadness. People who haven't been able to let themselves mourn over a great loss or have denied themselves a grieving period can turn their tears inward, so to speak. Chronic loose coughs and other types of lung congestion may also be the result of crying on the inside.

Do you need to allow yourself some crying time? A reflexology treatment may bring this release of emotions out in you. Choose a reflexologist you feel safe with. He or she will understand that reflexology can trigger the release of more than just physical toxins.

Asthma can also be associated with the feeling of being suffocated mentally or emotionally by someone in your environment. Is your boss smothering your creativity? Do you feel your roommate doesn't allow you to speak up or express your emotions? Do you think you're being held back because someone around you is overly protective? A holistic reflexology approach not only looks at the physical causes of illness, but takes into account other causes as well. Your lungs can give you some clues into what's going on in your emotional environment.

**Tip Toe**

Breathing clean air, aerobic exercise, deep-breathing exercises, refraining from smoking, taking certain respiratory herbs like lobelia and fenugreek, and wearing protective masks when dealing with chemicals all help protect your lungs. Reflexology can help by breaking up mucus deposits left in your lungs, making it easier for your body to expel any physical or emotional irritants.

# Sinus Up for Reflexology

The sinuses are the air passageways in the head located above the eyebrows, behind the eyes, and on either side of the nose. These little cavities are responsible for warming up the air we breathe before it goes into the lungs. The sinuses also have some filtering capabilities linked to the mucus membranes that transport mucus through small channels into the nasal cavity.

On the foot, the sinuses' reflex points are represented by the soft padding on all the toes. Squeezing the toes works these reflex points. On the hands, the finger pads represent the sinuses. You can also work on these by squeezing each finger.

The fingers and the toes all correlate to the zones and reflexes for the sinuses. Squeezing these when you have a sinus infection or sinus congestion may help you relieve the pain and pressure. Reflexology is not a substitute for fighting infection, but it can help you with discomfort and help boost your immune system to help you fight infection. And don't forget: when you're suffering from infection or your body is discharging mucus, be sure to keep up your fluid intake.

> **Foot Note**
>
> One of my clients once told me that my reflexology treatments were a draining experience. I was hurt until she clarified that her sinuses drained every time I worked on her!

## More Tips for the Stuffed-Up

You can also work the tips of the fingers and toes by squeezing them and holding each one individually until you notice the pain subsiding in your sinuses. If you're at home, you might want to put clamps on your toes or fingers to help alleviate the pain of a sinus infection. Just don't leave them on too long. Five minutes at a time is plenty!

In my experience, reflexology has worked instantaneous wonders for the chronically stuffed-up head. Along with asthma, I used to be one of those who pronounced my "M"s like "Ebb"s. If you can't relate, hold your nose and say the letter M—see what I "bean"?

If you're stuffed up from allergies but don't have an infection, reflexology can help relieve the congestion. Stimulate the following reflex points to help relieve head congestion:

- ◆ Eyes
- ◆ Ears
- ◆ Inner ears
- ◆ Sinuses

> **Tip Toe**
>
> You can make your own clamps to use on your fingers or toes to stimulate the sinus reflex points. Find some spring-loaded clothespins. Remove the wire, replace it with a rubber band, and voilà, instant clips! Put one on each toe or finger when you have allergy or sinus troubles.

I frequently see folks with sinus congestion from a head cold or allergies. Many times sinus congestion is released immediately after I begin working on them. This release has been described as a popping sensation followed by a relief of congestion. Working primarily on the padding of the foot just below the toes has helped in these conditions.

| Foot Note |
| --- |
| Allergies and asthma, bronchitis, and all ailments of the respiratory tract limit us in taking a full breath of life. It's wonderful to know that reflexology can be useful in changing these problems. Reflexology is safer than asthma and allergy medications and has no ill side effects. Reflexology used at home is as free as the air we breathe and may make a huge difference in how we feel! |

Generally, the left sinus reflexes correspond to the left foot and hand and vice versa. However, sometimes your experiences don't necessarily reflect this division. For example, when your sinuses are clogged and you work on your left sinus reflex area, you might not feel an instant draining of the left sinus. But when you begin to work on the right hand, the left sinus may begin to drain.

I think this has to do with a buildup of pressure from increasing the circulation when working with reflexology. Or it could be that sometimes it just takes time for the work on the other side to kick in, so to speak. This has happened to me over and over, and you might experience this for yourself, too.

# *Ears* to Having You Work on My Feet!

The ear reflexes are located on the padding of the ball of each foot just underneath the fourth and fifth toes. The eustachian tube is the tube that runs from the inner ear connecting it to the back of the throat. Its reflex area runs along the base of all the toes and up along the inner edge of the large toe on each foot.

The ear reflexes are on both hands and are located on the palms just below the ring and pinky fingers, and the eustachian tube reflex runs along the padding of the palm at the base of the fingers.

Clapping your hands vigorously can be considered a form of reflexology. Clapping is an easy way to affect most of the sinus areas on the hands. The fingertips are stimulated on one hand, and the eyes and ears of the other hand are stimulated simultaneously. You know what this means, don't you? When you see me at the next book signing, I expect a standing ovation!

The inner ear is associated with your sense of balance. If you have water on your eardrum due to some type of infection or fungus growth, or have excess wax in your ear, you can become dizzy or even experience *tinnitus*, or ringing in the ears.

The ears are an excellent area to work on when you have sinus troubles. The stimulation of reflexology treatments may help relieve a congested feeling in the head. Performing an *ear coning* after a reflexology treatment on someone whose ears are clogged is sure to make you a hero!

## def•i•ni•tion

Tinnitus is characterized by any noise, buzzing, or ringing in the ear. Causes of tinnitus may be excess ear wax, damage to the eardrum, Meniere's disease, or thinning blood due to overuse of aspirin or other drugs. Dr. Bernard Jensen also links tinnitus to a lack of magnesium. **Ear coning** or ear candling is an ancient healing therapy used to aid the ears and upper respiratory system. Ear coning is still used today as a gentle way to stimulate the body's circulation to the ear, which brings about the body's natural healing abilities. While having your ears coned, tiny ear reflex points around the ear opening are stimulated by the gentle pressure of the cone. These ear reflex points include primarily the throat and mouth, nose, and inner ear.

For those who have ear wax buildup, or any type of sinus problem, I like to work on the toes vigorously. This practice seems to break up and loosen old debris from the ear and upper sinus passages so the body's elimination channels can easily remove it. Some people claim I've changed their voice after a treatment followed by an ear coning. The only real difference is that they can hear themselves better.

# *Eyes* Can See Clearly Now

The eyes are wondrous, fascinating extensions of the brain that serve many functions. They deserve a whole book to themselves, but here I'm tying them in with the respiratory system.

The eyes receive information, and it's thought that they're also instruments for sending energy. And of course, the eyes provide us with the gift of sight. Because some of the sinus cavities are located close to the eyes, pressure buildup or sinus headaches can make your eyes ache or tear. When allergens are in the air, your eyes may itch and water to help reject these irritants.

> **Tip Toe**
>
> A body reflexology tip for the eyes: gently press in with your fingertips all around your eye sockets, looking for tight muscles. The pressure may create a popping sensation when the muscle releases. Loosening up these tightened muscles can bring a renewed vitality to tired eyes.

The eye reflex areas are located in the same area along the ball of each foot at the base of the toes near the ear reflexes. The eye points are the areas below the second and third toes. They're also found in the corresponding points on the hands, on each palm just under the pointer and middle fingers.

Respiratory troubles are not the only things that can cause eye problems. Diseases such as macular degeneration, night blindness, and glaucoma all have different causes, including malnutrition. Our habits can also increase our risk of certain eye diseases. For instance, smoking and overexposure to the sun can contribute to the development of cataracts. Tightening of the muscles surrounding the eyes sometimes causes near- and far-sightedness, which not only distorts the shape of the eye, causing vision inadequacies, but can also slow the amount of blood circulating to the eyes.

In the case of glaucoma, fluid and pressure buildup behind the eye can squeeze off the drainage ducts, preventing them from emptying properly.

Reflexology helps relax all muscles—including the eye muscles—and this may be a wonderful way to help relax muscles and improve circulation in general to the eyes, which may help prevent or even reverse eye disorders that are exacerbated by tension and stress. Whatever the cause of the eye problems, stimulating the eye reflex points on the feet and hands is a great natural and safe therapy you can use to help revitalize the eyes.

## The Least You Need to Know

◆ Reflexology can facilitate a cleansing process in the lungs and bronchials that can cause a person to cough up excess mucus after a treatment.

◆ Reflexology can play a role in helping asthmatics because of the relaxation it can bring to the bronchial tubes and the nervous system as a whole.

◆ The lungs are associated with grief. If you're not getting over your lung problems with natural therapies, ask yourself if you need to take time to grieve.

◆ Squeezing the fingers and the padding of the toes can sometimes work instantaneously to relieve sinus congestion, helping drain mucus to unclog a stuffed-up head and ears.

◆ Reflexology promotes overall muscle relaxation and sends healing energy and helps restore circulation to the eyes, which can help prevent vision problems.

# Chapter 13

# Give Me a "P": The Urinary System

## In This Chapter

◆ Learn the importance of the urinary system organs

◆ Locate the major urinary system reflexes on the feet and hands

◆ Understand some of the root causes of urinary troubles

◆ Learn some natural ways to correct urinary tract problems

My favorite radio commercial here in Boise is for a local plumbing company. Their motto is "A-1 Plumbing: We're the best place in town to take a leak."

Although you don't call a plumber if you have problems with your urinary system, you still have to take care of your body's "pipes." Your urinary system serves many more functions than just carrying off liquids from the body. Let's take a look at what your interesting internal plumbing does for you and see how you can take better care of it with reflexology, starting with locating the urinary system reflexes.

# Liquid Plumber

The urinary system serves as the body's plumbing system, and its organs, including the bladder, kidneys, and ureter, serve to eliminate liquid wastes from the system. The pipes also play a role in helping maintain proper fluid balance in the body, helping maintain salt balance, and keeping an acid/alkaline base balance in the bodily fluids.

> **Tip Toe**
>
> The recurrence of some types of kidney stones may be prevented by an adequate intake of magnesium. A few foods rich in magnesium are yellow cornmeal, bananas, nuts, soy, and rice polishings.

Do you have trouble with any of the following?

♦ Bladder infections

♦ Kidney infections

♦ Kidney stones

♦ Incontinence

♦ Edema

♦ Frequent urination

These are all troubles related to the urinary system. But before you call a plumber, let's try to find the cause of your troubles first!

There are many ways to support the urinary system, and reflexology is one of them.

*The hand reflexes for the urinary system. These reflexes are the same for the right hand.*

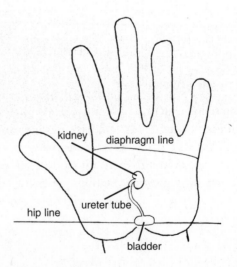

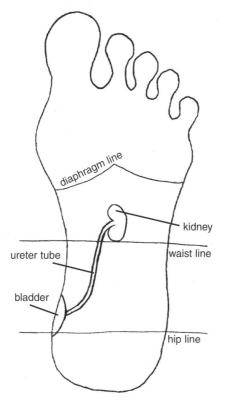

*The foot reflexes for the urinary system. These reflexes are the same for the right foot.*

# Fill 'Er Up: The Bladder

The urinary bladder is a closed sac composed of a smooth muscle coat that stores a liquid bodily waste called urine. The bladder holds this material until it tells you by nerve impulses that it's full. When this happens, you have the urge to urinate. When you do, the bladder then flattens and even becomes somewhat concave on the top and leans forward toward your lower abdomen. When it's full, the bladder becomes round, like a full balloon, and projects slightly upward.

The bladder reflex area is found on the sole of each foot along the medial, or inside, edge just slightly above the heel of each foot. You can

**Tread Lightly** _____

Ignoring your body's urge to urinate can weaken the bladder by stretching it. The stagnation may also make you more prone to bladder infections. So for bladder health, listen to the call of nature.

find this point by using your thumb to dig around that area. You'll know when you're on the bladder reflex because it will feel like a slightly hollow area, like it almost perfectly fits the tip of your thumb.

The bladder area on the hands can be found on the lower middle palm of both hands, just above the wrist. You can tell by feel where the bladder area in the hand is, also. The tip of your thumb should naturally fit right in this little intersection of the palm. Try this tip to make it easier to find:

- Lay the backside of your left hand flat, palm facing up.

- Pretend you're making a karate chop with your right hand directly to the base of the fingers of your left hand.

- Then touch your left thumb to your right palm. If you follow the natural diagonal movement of your thumb, it will land at the bottom middle of your other hand's palm.

- Your thumb will be pointing to the bladder area.

# Bladder Infections: A Bad Burn

If you have a bladder infection, you'll feel a pressure on the bladder to urinate even when the bladder is empty. When infections are bad, blood can be passed into the urine, and urination causes a painful burning sensation. Ouch!

I can attest to the fact that bladder infections can be extremely painful. Fortunately, I am also living proof that reflexology can help speed the healing of and even prevent bladder infections!

When I first began my reflexology training, I was getting bladder infections on a regular basis. When I found out where my bladder reflex point was, I went to town on it! I noticed even before I started manipulation on the bladder reflex point that the area was swollen and slightly red. When I first touched my bladder reflex point, I was amazed at how crunchy and tender the spot was.

To make a long story short, or a round bladder flat, every time I felt a bladder infection coming on, I worked deeply on my bladder reflex point. The area was always swollen and tender, and I worked on it until the tenderness subsided. The therapy worked! I got good at catching the beginning symptoms soon enough to work my reflex points, and my full-blown, painful bladder infections never manifested. I have only had one bladder infection since that first reflexology class 10 years ago!

> ⚷ **Tip Toe** _____
>
> For years, unsweetened cranberry juice has been used as a safe home remedy for bladder infections. Cranberries contain a group of compounds called proanthocyanidins, which are condensed tannins. Cranberries can also change the acidity level in the bladder. Both of these things are thought to prevent bacteria such as E. coli from attaching to and irritating the bladder lining. Drink lots of this juice, and lots of pure water when fighting off infection. Sugar may make your problem worse. If you don't like the taste of cranberry juice, try taking cranberry capsules instead.

Bladder infections can be related to chronic constipation. When your sewer system is backed up, the body has to deal with more toxins and fermentation than usual. The urinary system tries to deal with ridding the body of excess toxic wastes, which may lead to an infection. Therefore, it's a good idea to also work on your colon reflex areas when you're experiencing a bladder infection. Be sure you get cleaned out so your body has a chance to heal.

# Pintos or Kidneys?

The kidneys are small organs, reddish-brown in color, and shaped like—guess what?—a kidney bean. Most people have two kidneys, one on each side of the body located about midback, straddling the waistline.

The kidneys are responsible for filtering toxins, wastes, ingested water, and mineral salts out of the bloodstream. The kidneys are also responsible for regulating the acidity of the blood by excreting alkaline salts

> ⚷ **Tip Toe** _____
>
> The kidneys are important organs that serve many functions. They regulate body water and concentrations of electrolytes such as sodium, potassium, calcium, phosphorus, chloride, glucose, and amino acids. They aid in synthesizing vitamin D, hormones, and enzymes, and can even raise the oxygen-carrying capacity of the blood!

when necessary. Often, the left kidney is positioned up to an inch higher than the right kidney. The average adult's kidneys are about 4 to 5 inches long, about 2 inches thick, and weigh 4 to 6 ounces.

The kidneys serve important functions, including controlling water levels in the body. They also serve as filters of toxins and blood waste products contained in the liquids, foods, and air we take in.

The kidney reflex location is right in the center of the sole of the foot at about the middle of the waist line. The reflex can be found on each foot, one for each side. On each hand, the kidney reflex location is on the palm just about in the center.

## Drinking for Water Weight

When a person is carrying an excessive amount of water weight, the kidneys might not be functioning effectively enough to carry off the excess waste products or there might be a mineral imbalance resulting in water retention.

The body relies on a good supply of water to help it flush out waste products. Sometimes when we don't take in enough water, the body responds by holding on to water to protect it from *dehydration*. This is usually corrected by drinking at least eight glasses of water each day.

### def•i•ni•tion

Dehydration is the lack of water in body tissues. Lack of sufficient water intake, vomiting, diarrhea, and sweating can all be causes of dehydration. Symptoms may include great thirst, nausea, and exhaustion. If drinking plenty of water doesn't immediately correct the problem, sometimes water and salts need to be administered intravenously at an emergency room.

Along with reflexology treatments, drinking plenty of water helps your body release the water it's been hanging on to. This may take several weeks to accomplish, but after your body's cells understand that they'll be receiving enough water to keep the body balanced, they'll be able to let go of their stash.

## Sticks and Stones

Kidney stones are a product of built-up mineral salts called *calculus.* Passing kidney stones through the tiny ureter canal can be severely painful. If the stone gets stuck and blocks the flow of urine, surgery may be required.

The causes of kidney stones are generally the same as any problem with the urinary system, including the following:

- Too much protein in the diet

- Improper digestion

- Improper mineral intake

- Not drinking enough water

Lower back pain may disguise itself as kidney trouble or vice versa. If you have such pain, take this test to see if your lower back is bothering you or if it's your kidneys giving you problems. Stand up and have someone stand beside you to brace you when you do this exercise.

- Stand up straight and slowly lean backward.

- If you get a sharp sensation of discomfort, this could indicate that your lower spine is out of alignment and pinching a nerve.

- If the ache is still there but leaning back doesn't cause a sharp pain, your kidneys could be calling for some help.

To give your kidneys the help they need, first drink plenty of water. Parsley and juniper berries are excellent herbs that help the kidneys expel toxins. Hydrangea is used in the herbal world as a stone solvent and helps break down stones naturally. Avoid caffeine-containing products that may irritate the kidneys, and see your doctor if you suspect infection or a stone. And of course, work your kidney reflex areas!

If you have the feeling of a belt being cinched tightly around your waist, you could be experiencing a kidney infection. Work with the kidney reflex areas immediately, drink plenty of water, and get medical help right away! A serious kidney infection can be a life-threatening condition.

> **Tread Lightly**
>
> If you're experiencing a lot of back pain and general malaise along with a tension around your middle that feels like a belt being tightly cinched around your waist, you could be experiencing a kidney infection. In this case, drink plenty of water or parsley tea and work on your kidney reflex points on the way to your doctor's office!

## Getting in Balance

When you have high blood pressure, you should also take into account the health of your kidneys. The kidneys help keep your mineral salts in balance and, therefore, have a hand in regulating your blood pressure.

If you have high blood pressure, lower back pain, bags under your eyes, and a tendency to retain water, you fit the profile of someone who might have kidney trouble. The best thing you can do is to eliminate acid-forming foods from your diet, including coffee and red meats, and lower your cheese intake. Eat more raw green vegetables, and take a mineral supplement from nature such as alfalfa and liquid chlorophyll and colloidal minerals. Other supplements that may be helpful to the kidneys include vitamin D, B-complex, and l-glutamine. Drink much more water, cleanse the colon, and utilize reflexology every day until your blood pressure is regulated. After it's regulated, you can use reflexology less often to maintain your health.

# Urine Luck

While we're on the subject of releasing toxins, let's talk about urine. Urine is made up of water, urea, creatine, uric acid, and ammonia, among other things. These are all byproducts of digesting proteins. Anything that leaves an acid base in the body, such as heavy protein foods, stress, and physical exercise, can cause an overacidic body condition. Because part of the urinary system's job is to help maintain an acid/alkaline balance in the bloodstream, overacidity can put a strain on the kidneys and weaken the entire urinary system.

**Tread Lightly**

Ammonia is the end product of metabolizing protein. Too much protein can cause ammonia to rise in the body and make your kidneys work harder to keep you in balance. High-protein foods to avoid while suffering from kidney problems include most meats, nuts, beans, and dairy products. Eat more greens instead.

A chemical analysis of sweat shows that it has the same components as urine. The skin serves as a "third kidney." This is why you don't urinate as much in the summer as you do in the cold months. In the summertime, the skin makes up for eliminating the uric acid waste through perspiration. You also usually wear less clothing in the summertime and, therefore, the skin evaporates wastes more easily than in the winter, when you are heavily clad in long-sleeved shirts and socks.

If skin is underactive, uric acid, dead cells, and other impurities remain in the body. The other eliminative organs, therefore, have to work harder to pick up the slack. If skin isn't stimulated to do its job, eventually toxins are deposited back into tissues.

Sweating and dry skin brushing are two ways to stimulate the skin to eliminate and take a load off the kidneys. You can work up a sweat in a number of interesting ways, and I'll leave that up to you. Skin brushing might be new to you, however. Here's how to do it:

◆ Use a dry, vegetable bristle massage brush with a long handle. It's not an expensive brush. *Do not use nylon.*

◆ Use this brush first thing in the morning when you arise, before putting clothes on and before any bathing.

◆ Brush in either a circular or upward fashion, always toward the heart, all over the body except your face. Use a special facial brush for this more delicate skin.

It's important for you to support the urinary system by eating lots of alkaline-forming foods. Most fruits and all green vegetables and leafy greens such as lettuce, spinach, and parsley, as well as liquid chlorophyll are all good for this.

# Ureter–Always Wanted to Meet Her

The ureter tubes allow urine to flow down from the kidneys into the bladder. You have two ureter tubes, one for each kidney.

The reflex area for the ureter tubes is located on the sole of each foot and runs from the kidney area down to the bladder reflex. This is actually how the area can be worked. You can work your thumb down from the kidney, down the ureter, and end at the bladder.

The reflex area for the ureter tubes is also located on each hand (palm side) and also runs from the kidney area down to the bladder reflex.

I find that this area is one of the most sensitive parts of the foot, so start gently and see what the reaction is. Sometimes uric acid buildup can settle at the bottom of the nerve endings on the feet, and when reflexology treatments break up these crystals, the sensation can feel like you just stepped on a sharp rock!

Always drink plenty of water after a reflexology treatment, but especially if you find a lot of crunchies in the urinary reflexes. Your body will need extra water to help flush out any calcifications that may have been prompted to disperse. And after working on your urinary system reflexes and especially after any full reflexology session, try a hot Epsom salt bath (about 1 pint Epsom salts to a tub of hot water). This further aids in not only relaxing your muscles, but also aids the detoxification process through the skin and helps alkalize your entire system, which takes a burden off your kidneys.

## The Least You Need to Know

◆ Your urinary system not only filters waste products, but also serves to balance and help maintain the water, sodium, and other mineral levels in the body.

◆ When the body is overacidic due to stress, a high-protein diet, or poor digestion, the kidneys have to work harder to filter out the excess acid waste.

◆ High blood pressure can be due to the kidneys not functioning properly.

◆ The skin serves as a third kidney, so it's important to allow the skin to breathe and perspire by exposing it to fresh air and stimulation, such as skin brushing.

# Chapter 14

# The Heart of the Matter: The Circulatory System

## In This Chapter

◆ Learn about the main components of the circulatory system

◆ Find the heart reflexes on the foot and hand

◆ Understand how your blood works and how reflexology can help keep it moving

◆ See why reflexology helps in matters of the heart

We can't live without our hearts, although some of us live with our hearts on our sleeve! Heart and soul are sometimes considered the same thing. When we give and receive reflexology, we not only help the circulatory system, but also share good energy, which just may be a supplement the heart requires. Researchers are finding that many people live longer when they're paired up with a companion. So let's find out how we can be good to our hearts through our soles!

# Circulating Rumors and Other Things

The circulatory system consists of the blood, blood vessels, and the heart. It's the means by which the heart pumps blood through the veins and arteries. The circulatory system makes it possible for all the organs to receive nutrients, oxygen, and other substances necessary for sustaining life.

On a continual basis, oxidation and metabolism waste by-products are collected by the circulatory system and carried to the correct places for elimination or recycling. It's almost like our grocery stores' delivery trucks and our garbage trucks all traveling on the same road.

Circulatory system imbalances include the following:

- High or low blood pressure

- High cholesterol levels

- Heart attacks

- Strokes

- Broken blood vessels

- Irregular heartbeat

- Low or high blood count (which is also related to the liver)

- Mitral valve or other heart-related dysfunction

> **Tread Lightly**
>
> Signs of a heart attack include sudden and usually severe chest pain that may radiate through the arms and possibly the throat. If you're experiencing chest pain, you could be having a heart attack. *Call 911 (or your local emergency number) immediately!*

# Be Still My Heart

The heart is the major organ of your circulatory system. It rests in your chest cavity slightly left of center. The heart is a muscular, cone-shaped organ about the size of a clenched fist. Mechanically, it serves as a pump. It beats normally about 70 times per minute, powered by balanced nerve impulses and muscle contractions. Factors affecting the pulse rate include emotion, exercise, hormones, temperature, pain, and stress.

In foot and hand reflexology, the heart is really the only component of the circulatory system that's charted. Because your veins, arteries, and capillaries run throughout your body, you are sure to stimulate the entire circulatory system when you work on any parts of the feet or hands. The heart reflex area is found on the sole of the left foot and covers just about the entire ball of the foot.

On the hands, the heart area is found on the palm of the left hand and covers the area between the diaphragm line and the base of the fingers. More advanced charts may add the fourth and fifth fingers to the heart area as well. The pinky finger represents heart energy patterns, so it, too, can be worked as a heart reflex. See the illustrations of the left foot and hand so you know where to find your heart.

**Tip Toe**

The heart is predominately a potassium organ. Potassium is important in healing, aiding nerve synapses, vitality, preventing the formation of uric acid, and aiding hair growth. A mineral imbalance or potassium deficiency can lead to heart fluctuations, irregularities, and sometimes high blood pressure.

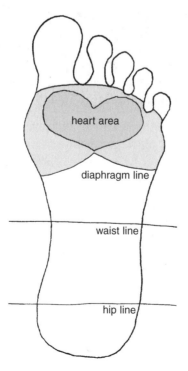

*The heart reflex on the left foot. You can also work the fourth and fifth toes to stimulate cardiac reflexes.*

heart area

diaphragm line

waist line

hip line

*The heart reflex on the left hand. You can also work the ring and pinky fingers to stimulate cardiac reflexes.*

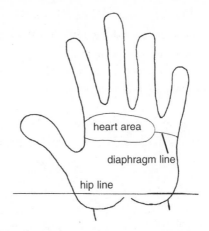

# Keep Circulating: Veins and Arteries

The veins are the channels of transportation for blood that carry deoxygenated blood and waste products to the heart. The veins and arteries are really the same type of transportation vessels, but they carry their goods in different directions.

The veins and arteries are not mapped out on the foot, but a vigorous reflexology treatment brings circulation down to the feet and hands and has a warming effect on them. If your feet are not warm and your toenails look pale, circulation is lacking to your extremities. Reflexology will help you restore circulation to your feet and hands.

Arteries are blood vessels that are responsible for carrying oxygenated blood from the lungs through the heart and then away from the heart to distribute blood to the rest of the body. Our arteries should be strong but elastic. Hardening of the arteries is known as *arteriosclerosis*, a chronic disease in which the arteries become thick and hard and lose their elasticity, resulting in impaired blood circulation. Symptoms may include the following:

- ◆ Cold hands and feet
- ◆ Blurred vision
- ◆ High blood pressure
- ◆ Difficulty thinking
- ◆ Difficulty breathing

**def•i•ni•tion**

**Arteriosclerosis** is a chronic disease in which the arteries become thick, hard, and lose their elasticity, resulting in impaired blood circulation.

Causes of arteriosclerosis have been linked to too much saturated fat in the diet; lack of aerobic exercise; and too much caffeine, salt, or alcohol in the diet.

## Warm Hands, Cold Heart?

It's a challenge to send good circulation to the extremities such as the feet and hands, because these areas are the farthest away from the trunk of the body where the heart "pump" is located. The body knows the most important organs to keep nourished and warm are contained in the head and trunk areas. Because blood warms your body, your blood tends to stay mostly in the center of your body, and your limbs are more subjected to outside temperatures than your core.

When outside temperatures are cold, blood tends to retract toward the middle of the body. This is a natural body function; it's only unnatural when someone has cold hands and feet all the time. This could mean their circulation isn't strong enough to get the warm blood out to the ends of the extremities. It could also mean they have low blood pressure or a low blood count.

Reflexology really comes in handy in these cases because outside stimulation of the feet and hands naturally brings blood to those areas, warming them up, nourishing the tissues, and flushing out accumulated toxins. Improved circulation through reflexology, therefore, can aid in healing the body.

> **Tip Toe**
>
> Reflexology actually stimulates the heart and all body parts through reflex action. It's believed that reflexology helps the body dissolve blood clots—working remotely, helping directly.

## Blood Pressure and Emotions

Our environment, emotions, and what and how we think can and do influence our blood pressure and even our cholesterol levels. Stress can raise both!

When seeking reflexology treatments for high blood pressure, it's important that you find a reflexologist who makes you feel safe and

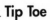

**Tip Toe**

You can find a professionally trained and certified reflexologist or even find approved reflexology schools and programs through such national organizations as the American Reflexology Certification Board (www.ARCB. net) or Reflexology Association of America (www. reflexology-usa.org).

comfortable and whose environment or touch doesn't stress you out. Seek a professionally certified reflexologist, because they should have already been trained in the importance of client comfort and the professional environment.

Reflexology, when executed properly, is incredibly relaxing, so having a reflexology session by someone you trust can have a direct effect on helping balance out your blood pressure. And who knows, maybe with weekly sessions of being de-stressed through reflexology, it might even have an effect on lowering cholesterol!

## Tiny Vessels: The Capillaries

Our blood capillaries are the tiniest vessels in our circulatory system. These delicate vessels are only one single cell thick! The capillaries allow an exchange of carbon dioxide, oxygen, salts, water, and other nutrients between the blood and the tissues.

Capillaries can be easily broken, and they cause redness on the surface of the skin where they're broken or weakened. Some causes of broken blood vessels or capillaries include the following:

◆ Tight clothing

◆ Standing on your feet too much without exercise

◆ Crossing your legs

◆ Tight shoes

◆ Excessive alcohol consumption

◆ Exposure to extreme temperatures

**Tip Toe**

Alcohol, food allergies, and exposure to extremes in temperature may aggravate broken blood capillaries, especially in the face. Avoid these things, and also always wear sunscreen.

- Excessive sun exposure

- Anything that rubs or injures the skin for a prolonged period of time

When working on someone whose capillaries break easily, explain to them that they might find some bruising on their lower legs after your treatments. Try not to work too deeply on them, and give them some tips on how to strengthen their capillary walls nutritionally. A component in grape seed extract and pine bark, for example, has been found to be a powerful antioxidant and has been shown to strengthen capillary walls.

# Blood, Sweat, and Tears

Our blood is made up of cells carried in a liquid substance called *blood plasma*. The average adult male has about 5 liters of blood in his body. The liver, spleen, and bone marrow all take part in the production and recycling of blood.

> **Tread Lightly**
>
> Beware of working too deeply on a person with a blood clot. The increased circulation may dislodge the clot and could cause a stroke! Of course, the same thing could happen to them if they were to walk barefoot through their front yard, but just be aware of the dangers when you're working with anyone with life-threatening illnesses. Be sure the person you're working on also understands the risks.

Blood not only carries nutrients and oxygen to other parts of the body, but it also carries toxins, especially when our sewer system (lower bowel) is backed up. Because the skin is the closest eliminatory organ to the blood, when it's overloaded with toxins, it throws toxins out through the skin.

This is when we get pimples, rashes, and boils, and our skin itches! If you're slathering zit cream on your face day and night, remember that most skin ailments are caused by the dirty condition of your blood, not necessarily your skin! So when rashes and other skin ailments pop up, look for reasons why the blood is toxic. Look first at the bowel.

When you have skin ailments, work on your bowel and liver reflex areas to help stimulate those organs. You'll be amazed what a good bowel and liver cleansing will do for your skin! An herbal cleansing won't hurt either. You might want to try herbalist Ivy Bridge's daily colon cleansing drink.

---

### Foot Note

Ivy Bridge's daily cleansing drink: blend ½ glass apple juice, 2 table-spoons each whole leaf aloe vera juice and liquid chlorophyll, and 1 teaspoon or 8 capsules of psyllium hulls. Drink immediately with 2 cap-sules cascara sagrada. Follow up with 8 ounces water. Take this first thing in the morning for 60 days. Then take this every other day for 2 months, and finally one to two times a week indefinitely. It also helps normalize overacidic conditions and lowers cholesterol. Ivy stresses adding a daily food enzyme supplement to this cleanser to break up undigested proteins left in the digestive tract. And be sure to drink 2 to 3 quarts of water daily to flush toxins from the body.

---

Reflexology sessions can positively affect the circulatory system by stimulating circulation, sending a healing signal to the heart, de-stressing us. Reflexology can even come in handy in an emergency such as a heart attack. All excellent reasons why everyone should know the basics of reflexology!

## The Least You Need to Know

◆ The heart is the main organ of the circulatory system.

◆ Giving reflexology to someone you love benefits their circulation.

◆ High blood pressure can be caused by environmental or emotional factors. Reflexology can help balance blood pressure by creating time to relax in a stress-free environment during treatments.

◆ Skin ailments can come from a buildup of waste products in the blood, which comes from a sluggish colon and liver. When dealing with skin problems, work the bowel and liver reflex points to stimulate cleansing.

# Chapter 15

# Sexy Stuff: The Glandular System

## In This Chapter

- ◆ Get to know your thyroid gland and its role in your life
- ◆ Note key symptoms that could signal glandular imbalance
- ◆ Consider the role of the gonads
- ◆ See how your hormones affect how you feel
- ◆ Locate the reproductive system and thyroid reflex areas

Have you ever heard the question "Is it hot in here, or is it me?" Well, if it is you, it just might be your glandular system in overdrive! The glandular system encompasses many glands serving many functions. This chapter gives you an overview of the glandular system, including the reproductive organs, the thyroid, and the pancreas.

# Sex and the Glands

Most of the reproductive glands are part of the endocrine system. All these glands work together as a team to keep your body in harmony. When the ovaries are surgically removed, for example, the adrenals and thyroid have to take over to try and maintain hormonal balance. (I discussed the adrenals in Chapter 11 because they're related to stress hormones. They're actually a part of the endocrine system and are intimately linked to the other glands in that system.)

The endocrine system consists of the following:

- Adrenals
- Ovaries/testes
- Thyroid
- Pancreas (part of it)

- Pituitary
- Parathyroids
- Thymus
- Pineal

Symptoms of glandular imbalance range as wide as the plains of Montana and run high and low depending on the over- or underactivity of a particular gland. Usually, glandular imbalances involve conditions such as the following:

- Irregular menstrual cycles
- PMS or irritability
- Infertility
- Unexplained weight gain or loss
- Adult acne
- Insomnia
- Lethargy, mild depression
- Racing heart
- Facial hair (in women)
- Hot flashes or feeling cold all the time

Well, now you know the worst, so let's get on with it. Take a look at the following figures to see the hand and foot reflexes for the reproductive glands, the thyroid, and the parathyroids.

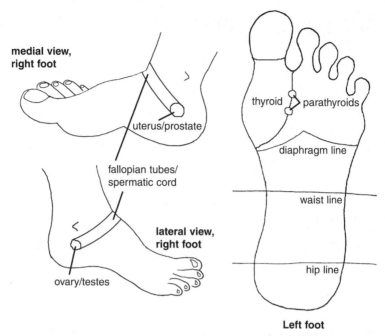

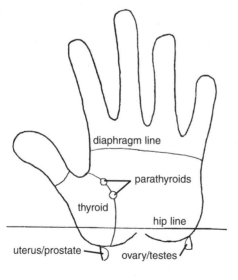

*The foot reflexes for the reproductive organs, thyroid, and parathyroids. The same reflexes are located on both feet.*

*The hand reflexes for the reproductive organs, thyroid, and parathyroids. These same reflexes are repeated on the palm of both hands.*

# The Thyroid—Metabolism Regulator

The thyroid is a small, pinkish gland that straddles the windpipe just below the Adam's apple in the throat. It's shaped kind of like a butterfly or a bat. Imagine a pink, fleshy butterfly wrapping its wings around your windpipe, and you can visualize your thyroid gland. The hormone-secreting thyroid is mostly responsible for your metabolism.

The thyroid area can be found on both feet and includes the area all around the base of the big toe (neck area) and the ball of the foot just below the big toe. You can press all around the base of your big toe with your thumb to work the tender spots. This therapy also helps loosen up your neck.

The thyroid area is found on both hands all along the padding of the palm at the base of the thumb.

The thyroid includes the *parathyroid glands*, which have a lot to do with keeping the calcium and phosphorus balance in the body. Their proper function is also important in poise and composure. The parathyroids are two pair of flattened tiny pieces of tissue on either side of the larynx on the thyroid gland. They're probably named parathyroids because there are two "pair a thyroids" on the thyroid! You can remember them as the spots on the ends of the wings of our pink thyroid butterfly.

## def•i•ni•tion

The **parathyroids** are two pair of flat, disc-shaped glands on each side of the thyroid gland. Think of them as the spots on the ends of the wings of the pink butterfly that represents the thyroid. The parathyroids help reg-ulate the calcium and phosphorus balance in the body. They are good reflex points to work on if you're dealing with arthritis and kidney stones.

The reflex areas for the parathyroids are two spots located together (one above the other) on the thyroid area between the webbing of the large toe and the second toe. I find these spots tender on many people. Press in on these tender spots, hold for 3 seconds, and repeat two more times. These areas are also located on both feet and hands.

On the hands, these parathyroid reflexes are found on the area of the padding of the thumb about in the middle edge of where the thyroid reflex runs through the palm. The thyroid area is easy to find on the hand because most of us have lines in the palm that correspond closely to this area. Look at your palm and see if you have a curved line that outlines the padded area of your thumb. If you do, you can use it as your landmark for where the thyroid and parathyroid areas are located.

## Thyroid Balancing Acts

Many problems are associated with a dysfunctional thyroid gland. Unfortunately, although medical tests can show thyroid blood tests to be in the normal range, you can still be suffering from a sluggish thyroid. Symptoms can include mild depression, dry skin, brittle nails, cold hands and feet, weight gain, changes in menstruation, and occasional migraines.

Thyroid receptors are not just in the thyroid but exist throughout the entire body. Some chemicals in our environment can bind with these thyroid receptors and slow the thyroid down or trigger an autoimmune response, which damages the thyroid. So it's important to try to avoid harsh chemicals and use more natural products in your home and on your body.

Of course, stress plays a role in lowering the thyroid energy, as well as hormone shifts such as perimenopause. When the thyroid is underactive due to prolonged stress and hormonal imbalance, reflexology can offer some stimulation and hopefully a bit of relief.

Reflexology cannot change nutrient deficiencies of the thyroid, of course. It can, however, utilize the pores on the soles of the feet, which are some of the largest pores on the body, to take in substances. For instance, in the case of an iodine deficiency that can cause enlargement of the thyroid, iodine could be applied to the soles of the feet. The pores are not only good for eliminating wastes from the body, but they also absorb some of what is applied to them. So please be careful what you step in!

> **Tip Toe**
>
> To determine if you have a sluggish thyroid, take this test: keep a thermometer by your bedside. Each morning for at least a week, as soon as you awake and before moving around, take your temperature and record the result. If the reading is an average of less than 97.6 degrees, you might suspect low thyroid activity.

## Seesaw or Balance Beam?

It's important to keep the thyroid in balance. The thyroid can become under- or overactive, and either extreme has its own symptoms. An overactive thyroid is known as *hyperthyroidism*, and a deficient or under-active thyroid is known as *hypothyroidism*.

Symptoms associated with an overactive thyroid include hyperactivity, a ferocious appetite, being underweight, nervousness, irritability, being emotionally imbalanced, and a racing heart. Eyes that appear as if they're popping out of the head could also be an indication of hyperthyroidism.

**def•i•ni•tion**

A **hyperthyroid** is an overactive thyroid. The hyperthyroid uses up iodine and other nutrients rapidly. A **hypothyroid** is a worn-out and underactive thyroid. It's usually too weak to produce the correct balance of thyroid hormones.

An underactive thyroid can slow you down. There are many indications that a person has low thyroid activity. Here's a fuller list of symptoms of hypothyroidism:

◆ Coarse hair, brittle and/or peeling fingernails, dry skin, hair loss

◆ Constipation

◆ Mild depression, loss of ability to concentrate, impaired memory, lethargy

◆ Difficult breathing

**Foot Note**

Hypothyroidism can be caused by continued exposure to low-dose radiation such as x-rays or mammograms, environmental pollution that depletes the body of vitamin A, and overuse of diet pills and other drugs. Women are eight times more likely to experience hypothyroidism than men.

◆ Excessive or irregular menstruation

◆ Weakness, general fatigue

◆ Headaches or migraines

◆ Low body temperature and/or low resting metabolic rate

◆ Deepening voice, slowed speech

◆ Pale lips, pallor of skin

◆ Poor vision

- Retarded growth in children and retarded mental development

- Puffy face, swelling of the eyelids, swollen feet and/or hands, thick tongue

- Unexplained or easy weight gain, especially around torso

The adrenal glands also help pick up slack for the thyroid, so if you think your thyroid is low, work those thyroid points and adrenal reflexes every day!

# Thyroid Be Done

The thyroid works in conjunction with the ovaries and some of the other glands, so it's a good idea to work with all the glands of the body if you suspect any problems with the thyroid. Reflexes to work on for thyroid trouble include the following:

- Thyroid area (along the ball of the foot under and around the neck of the large toe)

- Parathyroids

- Pineal gland

- Pituitary gland

- Ovaries

Because reflexology helps the body do what it's supposed to do naturally, stimulating the thyroid reflexes cannot damage the functioning of the organ. You can only help achieve balance. So don't worry about over-stimulating the thyroid with reflexology. Natural therapies don't cause this kind of reaction.

> **Foot Note**
>
> In glandular body typing, the thyroid body type is tall and thin with long fingers, arms, and neck. When overweight, these people hold the weight around their middle section and crave carbohydrate foods such as cookies and pastries. Thyroid types tend to be emotional and like to express themselves.

# The Gonads: By Dr. Phil D. Glanz

The reproductive organs do more than just help us procreate, although they are not necessary for our own survival. The ovaries and testes are parts of the glandular system that take their commands from the pituitary gland in the brain. (See—sex really is mostly in the head!)

Hormonal messages from the gonads command our sexual response, control hair growth, regulate menstrual cycles, keep the skin luminous, and give us a sparkle in our eyes. Imbalances in the reproductive organs can show themselves in the following ways:

- Cramps
- Hot flashes
- PMS
- Miscarriages
- Menstrual irregularities
- Ectopic pregnancies
- Infertility
- Frigidity

The uterus and prostate glands are also part of our reproductive system. Sometimes women who experience imbalances, or even cancerous conditions, in the reproductive organs have a radical surgery called a *hysterectomy*. *Hyster* comes from the Greek word *huster*, for womb. *Ectomy* is to remove something surgically. In the late 1800s, PMS was referred to as "hysterics" by some medical doctors.

The removal of the ovaries may plunge women into *menopause*, where the female body stops producing eggs for procreation. Reflexology can help you through menopausal symptoms by stimulating the balance of the other *endocrine glands* to make up for the lost ovary functions.

## def•i•ni•tion

A **hysterectomy** is the removal of a woman's uterus. **Menopause** is when a woman's ovaries stop producing eggs. The ovaries discontinue their hormone production, which can lead to dry skin, emotional instability, hot flashes, and heart palpitations. **Endocrine glands** are ductless glands that manufacture hormones and secrete them directly into the bloodstream. Endocrine glands include the pituitary, thyroid, parathyroid, adrenals, ovaries, testes, and part of the pancreas.

## Get Over Being *Teste* with Me!

*Ovaries* are two almond-shaped glands about an inch long located on the right and left sides of the pelvic area in females. These little glands are responsible for helping shape the female body, regulating the menstrual cycle, producing eggs (ova) for making babies, keeping the skin supple, and helping keep the calcium and other minerals in the body in balance.

The *testes* are two small, round glands each held in a saclike pouch located on the outside of a man's body. They are responsible for the production of hormones and for sperm storage. The hormones produced by the testes help in the construction of the structural system and are also responsible for mental attitudes and aggressiveness.

The reflex location for the ovaries and testes are the same on each foot. The ovary/testes spot is a small, round spot found at just about the center of the flat part of the outside of the heel, just below the ankle bone. Using your thumb or pointer finger to find this spot, you'll find somewhat of an indentation. This spot should not be overworked and is usually tender on everyone. Press on this spot for 3 seconds, release, and then repeat two more times.

On each hand, the ovary/testes reflex is located on the inside of the wrists on the pinky finger side, just below the heel of the hand. The same goes for both hands.

___ **Tip Toe** ___

A good way to remember the location of the ovary reflex is to remember your o's: the **o**vary/testicle reflex point is located on the **o**utside of each heel. The ovary and testes reflexes are interchangeable depending on the sex of the person you're working on. Remember "Get over being *teste* with me!" to remind you that the points are the same.

# PMS: Calming the Beast Within

One of the most widely studied uses of reflexology has been for relieving symptoms of PMS, or premenstrual syndrome. The results have been positive. Reflexology seems to help lessen severe symptoms of PMS through relaxation and stimulation of endorphins. Reflexology can also help with the pain associated with cramping before and during menstruation.

Some specific symptoms of PMS include the following:

♦ Mood swings

♦ Tension

- Irritability
- Bloating
- Headaches

Usually hormones are on a rampage, which can make a woman feel like she's out of control. Because the pituitary gland (in the brain) is responsible for sending hormonal messages to the rest of the body, it makes sense to stimulate this point when suffering from PMS or to stimulate this point on someone else who is experiencing PMS symptoms. Talk about making your point!

To ease the tension associated with PMS, work all along the brain and spinal cord areas to help relax all the muscles in the body. Utilize the relaxation and stretching techniques you learned earlier in this book. Of course, you should always work the ovary and uterus areas when dealing with any type of female issues.

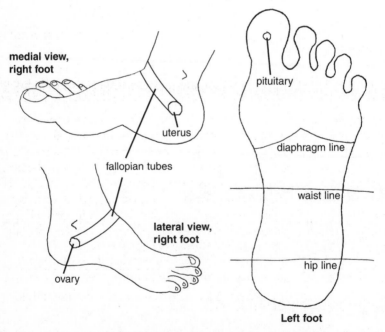

*Menstrual trouble reflex points. Working these spots on both feet has helped many women balance cycles and alleviate pain associated with menstrual cramps.*

Working the top of the foot (the opposite of the ball of the foot) can also prove useful for lessening tenderness in the breasts during PMS. To work the chest reflex areas, you can squeeze the webbing between all the metatarsals in the feet and hands.

Here's a summary of the points you can work on for PMS, so you can find them in a hurry:

♦ Pituitary (helps with water retention and regulating hormones)

♦ Brain (calms nerves and improves circulation)

♦ Spinal cord (calms nerves and brings out serotonin)

♦ Ovary (regulates hormones)

♦ Uterus (can ease contractions)

♦ Fallopian tube (relaxes pain in pelvic area)

♦ Chest area (opposite lymphatics on top of foot, work by squeezing webbing between metatarsals)

A wonderful technique for relieving menstrual cramps with reflexology is shown in Chapter 6.

| Foot Note |
|---|
| The gonadal body shape is a typical shape among women and, in rare cases, men. The gonadal, or reproductive, body type carries excess body weight in the hips, butt, and outer thighs, although their tummies are usually taut. This type is smaller on top than on bottom, similar to a pear shape, and have long, slender necks, smaller feet, and small ankles and wrists but are tallish. These people are attracted to rich, creamy foods; tend to be creative; crave affection; and have "rich" tastes. If you're a gonadal, stimulate your pituitary, pineal, and thyroid glands to stay balanced. Also, stay away from fatty foods, and eat more fruits and vegetables. |

## Uterus on to Prostate Health

The *uterus*, also known as the womb, is a pear-shaped organ suspended in the pelvic cavity that is specialized to allow an embryo to become implanted in its inner wall and subsequently to nourish the growing fetus. Problems with the uterus include the following:

- Miscarriages

- Endometriosis

- Cramps

- Hemorrhages

- Adult acne

**Foot Note**

A 1994 Danish study of reflexology's effect on infertility showed that of the 61 "infertile" women in the study, 15 percent became pregnant. The ones who didn't get pregnant showed positive effects with other menstrual cycle–related problems.

The *prostate* gland is a male accessory sex gland located just below the bladder. Its purpose is to secrete an alkaline fluid as part of the semen. The prostate gland is shaped like a donut, wrapping itself around the proximal end of the urethra snug up against the urinary bladder's exit.

Problems with the prostate often involve enlargement of the gland, putting undue stress against the neck of the bladder and impairing urination. This usually occurs in older men but can be managed and may be prevented with a holistically enhanced lifestyle that includes reflexology. Along with reflexology, the mineral zinc and the herb saw palmetto have been used to help shrink the prostate gland.

As the ovary and testes share the same reflex spot, so do the uterus and prostate. These points can be found on the inside middle of each heel, just below the ankle bone. Press and hold this point for 3 seconds, release, and repeat two more times. This is usually a tender spot on both males and females.

**Tread Lightly**

Prostate trouble is one of the most common ailments among middle-aged men. By age 50, 20 percent of American men have enlarged prostates, and by age 60, more than 50 percent do. (Statistics taken from Dr. Bernard Jensen's *Chemistry of Man* [Bernard Jensen, 1983].) Therefore, men should get regular prostate checkups after age 40.

The prostate/uterus reflexes can also be found on the inside of the wrist, just below the bottom joint of each thumb.

This is the point to work if someone is dealing with prostate trouble and waking up in the middle of the night to urinate. For women, this spot can be held when experiencing menstrual cramps or when in labor to help relax the uterus.

## Doing Some Tubing

One other reflex area that deserves a special mention under the reproductive system includes the fallopian tubes/spermatic cord reflex. The fallopian tubes are found in the female body and lead an egg (ovum) from the ovaries to the uterus for fertilization. Women own a pair of these tubes, one from each ovary, that come together at the uterus. The spermatic cord in men is the cord that runs from the abdominal cavity to the testicles.

The reflexes for these areas are located on both feet, running over the top of the foot from ankle to ankle, kind of like a strap that connects the uterus/prostate point to the ovary/testes spot. You can work this area in many ways, including finger and thumb walking (see Chapter 5) or by stimulating the area with a special rotation move (shown in Chapter 6).

The hand reflexes for these areas are not shown on my charts because they're located around the front part of the wrist. But when you work around the base of your hands, all around the wrist areas, you are stimulating your fallopian tubes/spermatic cord reflexes.

# Dealing with Diabetes

All right, so the pancreas isn't exactly sexy. Part of it does function in the body's glandular system, however, so I'm discussing it here for good measure.

I've worked with a handful of clients who had adult onset diabetes, a metabolic disorder that begins in the pancreas. Coincidence or not, after working with these people, not only did they feel better, but at least one of them was able to lower the amount of insulin she was required to take. Another client was on two types of insulin and was able to eliminate one of them with regular reflexology sessions!

Of course, this was done under the direction of their physicians. Both these women felt that their improvement was a testimonial to the fact that natural therapies can help the body work better. This also shows how reflexology can not only be a preventative or an alternative therapy, but also a complementary therapy to regular medical care.

Both of these diabetic women were on several medications during their treatments with me. The natural therapy, along with medical care, helped them recover and lessened their requirement for some medications.

## How Sweet It Isn't

Let's take a closer look at what diabetes is all about. *Diabetes mellitus* is the medical term for what most of us commonly call diabetes. It's a disorder of carbohydrate metabolism in which sugars in the body are not oxidized to produce energy due to lack of the pancreatic hormone insulin or because of the body's resistance to insulin.

## def•i•ni•tion

> **Diabetes mellitus** is a disorder of carbohydrate metabolism in which sugars in the body are not oxidized to produce energy due to lack of pancreatic insulin. Symptoms of diabetes include excessive thirst, sugar in the urine, and poor digestion. Complications can include poor circulation leading to slow healing, poor eyesight, weight gain, and coma if insulin and diet are not regulated.

The accumulation of sugar leads to its appearance in the blood, or *hyperglycemia*, which literally means high blood sugar. Symptoms include thirst, weight gain or loss, and the excessive production of urine. The use of fats as an alternative source of energy leads to disturbances of the acid/alkaline balance in the body and can cause *ketosis*, the imbalance of fat metabolism. If left untreated, diabetes can eventually lead to convulsions and even diabetic coma.

Long-term complications of diabetes include thickening of the arteries, which can affect the eyes. Other effects include circulation problems that can manifest as slow wound healing. This is probably due to the fact that the blood supply to the wounded area is decreased due to a sluggish circulatory system.

This is another reason why reflexology can be such a great therapy for people who suffer with diabetes. Reflexology stimulates circulation, which is necessary in healing wounds and can help get the blood supply moving and to the extremities, such as the hands and feet.

## Back in Circulation

Because of poor circulation associated with diabetes, several areas of the body are affected by the disease. The entire urinary system is affected, because the body is trying to rid itself of excess acid wastes. The eyes can also be troubled due to a lack of circulation. The adrenals are also affected, as well as the pancreas and the digestive system.

When working on someone who suffers from diabetes, work the areas that are most tender, as usual, but be sure you don't skip the following important areas:

- ◆ Eyes*
- ◆ Spleen
- ◆ Liver
- ◆ Pancreas*

- ◆ Stomach
- ◆ Adrenals
- ◆ Urinary system
- ◆ Kidneys*

The reflex areas marked with an asterisk (*) are the three *most important* areas to work for diabetes. Reflexology won't necessarily lower blood sugar levels, but it can help balance the glands and increase circulation. Increasing a diabetic's circulation can help their body speed up the healing process and help them get blood moving up to the head where it can nourish the eyes!

---

### Foot Note

A 1984 Danish study showed a clear increase in blood flow in the subject's body following reflexology treatments. Pictures taken with infrared rays, which can show changes in heat loss, showed the increased blood flow. It's assumed that the improved circulation achieved through reflexology treatments increased the oxygen supply to the brain (blood carries nourishing oxygen).

## The Least You Need to Know

◆ The reproductive system and glandular system, for our purposes here, include the ovaries or testes, uterus or prostate, thyroid and parathyroids, and fallopian tubes or spermatic cord.

◆ The thyroid regulates metabolism. A slow metabolism could mean an underactive thyroid.

◆ The ovary and testes areas are tender on most people and should not be overworked.

◆ The uterus and prostate reflexes are also tender spots, and moderate manipulation of this point may benefit menstrual cramps and/or prostate enlargement.

◆ A complication of diabetes is decreased blood flow to the extremities. Reflexology can help by increasing circulation throughout the body.

# Chapter 16

# A Psychological Workout

## In This Chapter

- ◆ Discover the ways reflexology can help the nervous system
- ◆ See how reflexology helps with insomnia
- ◆ Learn which reflexes may be helpful to work for psychological and nervous system disorders
- ◆ Find out how reflexology can calm nausea

The central nervous system, as you'll remember from the discussion in Chapter 11, is the highway that carries all the messages for all the body processes and functions. As long as you're not under anesthesia, the nervous system is aware of everything that goes on in the body. Reflexology is great for relaxing the nerves and balancing glandular secretions and can help with disorders of the nervous system.

In this chapter, I have included both nervous system disorders and psychological disorders. These may include the following:

◆ Bipolar (or manic-depressive) disorder

◆ Severe stress-related conditions

◆ Parkinson's disease

◆ Multiple sclerosis

◆ Some addictions

◆ Insomnia

◆ Attention deficit disorder (ADD)

This chapter highlights a few imbalances directly related to excessive stress or worry and shows you how to help yourself or others with reflexology sessions. I'll specifically discuss insomnia, bipolar disorder, nausea from nervous tension, and ADD. You'll see how others have been helped with these problems through reflexology.

# Rock-a-Bye Baby

When I covered the nervous system in Chapter 11, I discussed the pineal gland and its production of melatonin, a hormone nicknamed "the sleep hormone" or the "anti-aging hormone."

Melatonin is the chemical messenger our body manufactures to make us feel tired and help us go to sleep. As we age, our pineal gland produces less and less of this hormone. Other things may interfere with melatonin production, such as hormone therapy and the ingestion of alcohol and some drugs.

**def•i•ni•tion**

**Insomnia** is the inability to fall asleep or to remain asleep for an adequate length of time.

*Insomnia* can occur when the pineal gland is not producing enough melatonin. Insomnia has many other causes, including worry or high stress, blood sugar imbalances, thyroid imbalance, side effects of drugs or prescription medications, or the use of legal or illegal stimulants.

# When Counting Sheep Doesn't Work

Reflexology can be very helpful for those with insomnia. It's best that someone with insomnia have another person work on them to help with this problem. Working to put yourself to sleep can be difficult.

If you create the right atmosphere for your insomniac subject, making sure they're comfortable and feel secure, they may just fall asleep while you work on them! This has happened to me several times and is a great compliment to the reflexologist.

The main reflex points to work on an insomniac are:

◆ Pineal

◆ Brain

◆ Adrenals

◆ Solar plexus

◆ Thyroid and parathyroid

Start with the pineal gland reflex, located on each large toe and thumb. This gland may be sleeping itself and not producing enough of the invaluable melatonin hormone! Stimulate this point three times on each large toe and also on each thumb.

You'll know when you stimulate the point by the feeling of electric shock your partner will feel when you find it (see Chapter 11 for details). Ask your partner for feedback when you're trying to find this point. Most people jump when the point is correctly stimulated, although not everyone responds so outwardly.

Also be sure you work the entire brain area (all along the tops of each toe and fingertip) when a person complains of insomnia. In addition, all the relaxation techniques, such as the stretching and rotating techniques, help the body relax.

The adrenals may be weakened because of stress so they should also be reflexed. Be sure to also work the thyroid and parathyroids, as an imbalance of these glands affects metabolism and can be the cause of insomnia. The solar plexus is a new area I haven't covered yet, but it's key in relaxing the body, nerves, and mind, so I cover it in more detail next.

# A Bundle of Nerves

Many people who have insomnia are worriers, so be sure to work the solar plexus reflex in the feet and hands. The *solar plexus* is found right in the middle of the upper half of the trunk of the body, where the ribcage comes together about at the stomach level in front of the diaphragm. See the full reflexology charts in Chapter 1 to find the reflex location for the solar plexus. You will see that it is centered in the middle of the diaphragm line on both the hands and feet. The solar plexus is a great network of nerves that goes out to all parts of the abdominal cavity and has sometimes been called the abdominal brain. It's affected by stress, especially worry.

**def•i•ni•tion**

The **solar plexus** is an area found right in the middle where the rib cage comes together about at the stomach level in front of the diaphragm. It is a great network of nerves that goes out to all parts of the abdominal cavity.

When a person is worried or stressed, stimulating the solar plexus reflex can make them jump off your table! Be sure to warn the recipient before you stimulate their solar plexus, especially if they are worriers or have insomnia. Then follow these steps:

**Tip Toe**

For a variation on this solar plexus technique, use both hands, one on each foot at the same time for relaxation at the end of the session. Try both ways and choose the one that's most effective for you.

◆ Grip the foot as shown in the following photo. Or you can work on two feet at the same time if you prefer for an all-over rush!

◆ Find the indentation in the middle of the base of the ball of the foot (feet) just under the diaphragm (see the reflexology chart in Chapter 1).

◆ Ask the person to take a deep breath. If you like, you can take a deep breath with them to guide them. Press in and slightly upward with your thumb for 3 seconds while your partner holds their breath.

◆ Have your partner exhale while you slowly release pressure on the spot and pull the feet (foot) toward you. Do not remove your thumb(s) from contact with the spot; just relax the pressure.

◆ Repeat the stimulation of this point a total of three times.

You can go deeper each time you work this reflex according to the tolerance of your partner. Afterward, they should feel invigorated and relaxed.

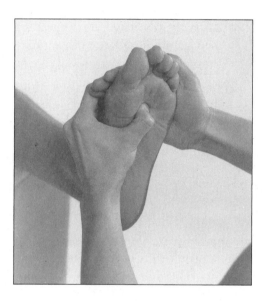

*Stimulating the solar plexus on one foot using one hand. For a variation, stimulate each solar plexus reflex simultaneously.*

# Leveling Out the Highs and Lows

*Bipolar disorder* is a severe mental illness usually caused by a chemical imbalance. The severity of this disorder varies, but its main characteristics are severe depression followed by mania (excitability). The episodes can be precipitated by emotionally upsetting events, but the reactions are often out of proportion to the causes.

The disease can be genetically inherited, but the full expression can be altered by environmental factors.

**def•i•ni•tion**

> **Bipolar disorder** is a severe mental illness characterized by severe depression followed by bouts of mania. Mania takes the form of obsession, compulsion, or an exaggerated feeling of euphoria.

I have seen many people with bipolar disorder come to a manageable balance with the addition of an integrated and holistic approach that includes reflexology, nutritional supplementation, and psychotherapy. I am amazed and encouraged at the progress I have seen my clients experience. Reflexology has played a role in helping these people facilitate more balance in their lives and many have been able to work with their prescribing physicians to get off of or at least lower their dosage of the psychotropic drugs used to treat this disorder.

Such a serious illness should always be addressed with more than reflexology; however, reflexology can assist hormonal and biochemical harmony and, therefore, may help the chemical imbalance of the brain.

Sometimes when in their manic state, people with bipolar disorder experience insomnia. Encourage relaxing reflexology sessions. With bipolar disorder, working the following reflexes aids in glandular and nervous system balance, and the relaxation techniques soothe the mind:

◆ Brain

◆ Spinal column

◆ Adrenals

◆ Solar plexus

◆ Pineal

◆ Pituitary

I have seen clients relax when they're in a manic state as a response to reflexology. I have also seen these people lift from their depression during a reflexology session. With regular sessions, these people begin to level out their highs and lows and regain a sense of stability.

---

### Foot Note

Although bipolar disorder is a chemical imbalance, I have seen a difference in those who have been brave enough to face the illness, actively take part in their recovery, and choose to be more conscious of their behaviors. I have seen some people make startling progress with natural therapies to supplement their traditional psychotherapy or other counseling sessions. Responsibility is empowering and can help anyone in their progress toward good health.

# A Look at ADD

Many children suffer from *attention deficit disorder* (*ADD*). The problems associated with ADD include an inability to focus attention on routine activities. Some have high frustration and choose to express themselves in violent outbursts. Others seem to not be able to sit still.

Adults suffering from this disorder may not necessarily show it outwardly as "misbehavior." In fact, these people often make great business entrepreneurs, as their overactive mental states can help breed creativity. Not only that, but adult sufferers of ADD usually have the drive to work ridiculous hours to make their businesses successful. The danger in this type of behavior is that running in overdrive all the time puts a burden on the adrenals and can lead to adrenal fatigue or exhaustion.

Reflexology has its place in working with hyperactive children and adults. Specific reflex points to work on for those who suffer from problems concentrating or who feel or appear hyper include the following:

◆ Brain

◆ Adrenals

◆ Central nervous system (spine and brain)

◆ Pineal gland

◆ Pancreas

Many children with food allergies or blood sugar imbalances suffer with ADD, and these possibilities should be investigated. In the meantime, working the reflex points to help the glands involved doesn't hurt and will likely prove useful.

---

### Foot Note

An ADD adult may run him- or herself into the ground and neglect family or friendships. Based on this behavior, many make too many promises that are impossible to follow through with. Needless to say, life works best for us in balance. Entrepreneurs with ADD may have great start-up businesses, but if they don't get their disorder under control, they might be better off selling their businesses before employees or the businesses suffer any damage.

# Calming Things Down

Feeling nauseated because of psychological or nervous system disorders is common. The brain plays a key role in making us feel sick or well, whether it's because of real or perceived threats that make us tense. When we relax the nerves, other symptoms that are caused by nerves, such as nausea, can be alleviated.

Reflexology makes a great therapy for children who are fussy but are too young to tell you what's wrong. I've seen car sickness alleviated with the use of reflexology. If you have someone in the car with you who can work on the child, ask them to press some reflexology buttons on the child's hands. If a carsick child is old enough, you can instruct them how to perform reflexology on themselves.

## Push My Nausea Button

Dizziness usually causes nausea. Dizziness, or the sense of losing balance, comes from sensations in our inner ear. Therefore, the inner ear reflex points are excellent areas to work for children (or adults) experiencing car, air, or sea sickness, or anything that involves a continuous rocking motion.

You can also work the stomach reflex in the hand, which aids a sick stomach. And finally, you can try the button for nausea by renowned foot, hand, and *body reflexologist* as well as author, Mildred Carter. Mildred says this "nausea button" is located on the inside of the wrist, between the two large tendons, found about three fingers from the wrist.

It may take a constant pressure for up to 20 minutes on this spot before relief is experienced. You may have seen bracelets claiming to relieve motion sickness; these bracelets are nothing more than elastic bands with a small "pea" that is placed on this reflex point.

**def•i•ni•tion**

**Body reflexology** is similar to foot and hand reflexology, but the reflexes are found over the entire body, not just the feet and hands.

Reflexology points helpful for nausea include:

♦ Inner ear

♦ Stomach

♦ Nausea button

♦ Spine

## Go to Sleep My Little Baby

Car sickness, or just plain old car grouchiness, can be cured with reflexology fairly quickly, as this story about a 9-month-old baby reveals.

Some years ago while visiting some friends and clients in Georgia, I had the privilege of sitting in the backseat next to my friend's 9-month-old baby boy for a 3-hour car trip.

Being a bit road weary myself and not knowing how to deal with children, I was not particularly delighted with the situation, especially because the boy had just discovered how to make long, loud noises with his throat and was fascinated with his ability to sound like a lawn mower running out of gas!

**Tip Toe**

The relaxing benefits of reflexology often put a baby or young child to sleep in the car, which makes them unaware of their car sickness or boredom!

After he got bored with his verbal experimentation, he decided he was grouchy. He began fussing and squirming in his car seat and began to whine quite loudly. In a desperate attempt to save my own sanity, I took his little hand in mine and began working his reflexes. In less than 3 minutes (and let me tell you I was counting!) the little bugger had his eyes closed and was quickly falling asleep.

The funniest thing about this story is that as I finished working one finger, he would stretch out the next finger as if to say, "Okay, now do this one!" The next 2½ hours were peaceful bliss for both of us! Reflexology to the rescue once again.

# Care with Compassion

As you've learned, although reflexology can be used as a self-help technique, when administered by another person, reflexology can be a mind-, body-, and soul-healing experience. Psychological disorders are complicated illnesses, but reflexology works by sharing compassion, too. It not only balances the glands, but may facilitate emotional release for folks dealing with emotional trauma or pain.

They say that making up your mind is 90 percent of anything you do. Maybe some psychological or chemical disorders and even nervous system disorders cannot be "cured," but they can certainly be managed to make them easier to live with. Sometimes just making the conscious decision to incorporate a natural healing therapy, such as regular reflexology treatments, into your life is a positive affirmation toward better management of your illnesses.

Your emotions have a tremendous impact on your health and should not be overlooked when you're looking for the causes of disease. The power of the mind is incredible and plays a big role in creating illness as well as health. An example of this is seen in cases where people suffering from multiple-personality disorder who have full-blown diabetes or other physical illnesses in one personality have absolutely normal body chemistry with no signs of physical disease in another!

But you must take care of the physical cause of any imbalance or illness first. Your emotions cannot correct a mineral imbalance, for instance, so you always need to look at where the environmental or nutritional voids exist first and work to correct the problem from there.

So for whole health, remember to think physically first and remove the possible causes of your problems. Then work on any emotional or spiritual connections and keep a positive attitude and mind-set to keep yourself healthy!

## The Least You Need to Know

◆ The solar plexus reflex on both hands and feet is the best reflex to work on when you're under a great deal of stress or worry.

- The pineal gland manufactures the hormone melatonin. It may be helpful to stimulate the pineal gland reflex if you have insomnia.

- Work the inner ear and stomach reflexes if you're experiencing nausea or car sickness.

- Fussy babies can quickly be relaxed with reflexology.

- Reflexology facilitates relaxation for the body, mind, and soul, making it an excellent remedy for nervous system and psychological disorders.

# Out of Step: Identifying (and Avoiding) Foot Problems

I've talked a lot about how to practice reflexology on someone in a general sense. Now let's learn how to read a foot! In a way it's like palm reading, but instead of the palm, you read the sole.

When you start working on other people's feet, you will naturally be exposed to many different types of foot problems. Remember, you are not a foot doctor, so I won't be getting into diagnosis—but it would be to your advantage, as well as your subject's, to know how to recognize some of the foot ailments you're going to see.

In Part 4, you learn some of the extras that can make your sessions more holistic and keep your friends and family members coming back for more!

# 17

# Finding Balance: The Elemental Foot

## In This Chapter

- ◆ Discover how to relate the condition of the foot to the four elements
- ◆ Understand some imbalances and what might cause them
- ◆ Learn how to best handle imbalances in foot conditions
- ◆ See how feet reflect imbalance in the rest of the body

Learning reflexology can be an interesting journey, because you might work with many different types of people one-on-one and see many different feet. With some experience, you'll begin to make associations with conditions of the feet and the condition of a person. You might also get to understand more about the four elements of earth, fire, water, and air and the balance they serve in all aspects of our lives. Let's take a closer look at how observing the feet can help the thoughtful observer learn something about the foot owner.

# The Four Elements

Air, fire, water, and earth make up all four basic elements on our planet. Nothing can exist without all four present, and you need a balance of each element in your life for health. The world could not exist without all the elements working together:

◆ The sun (fire) to provide light and heat

◆ The air to breathe

◆ The water to drink

◆ The earth to give us a place to stand and provide structure and supply an element from which to grow food

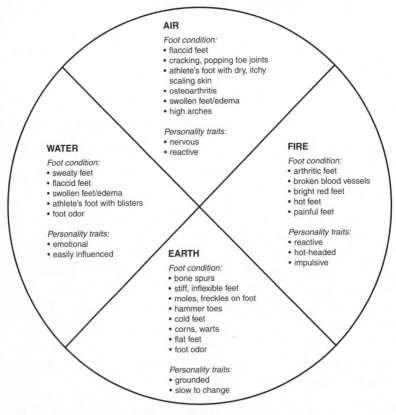

*This chart shows some foot conditions associated with each element. The condition is caused by an overabundance of the element. Personality traits of each element are also noted and are discussed in more detail in Chapter 19.*

When you understand how the elements interact with each other, you're better able to discover an appropriate solution. The four-element model is used to teach a philosophical way of seeing the elements in everything we do. In this chapter, we look at various conditions of the feet and see how they relate to the four-element model. You also learn how the model can help deal with an imbalance of the elements in the body.

Here's an example of using the four-elements to find a balance: too much fire causes hot, dry conditions. What's better to cool off a hot, dry condition than a little cool water? Keep the opposing type of energies and how they affect each other in mind as you use your four-element philosophy.

# Air: Snap, Crackle, and Pop

Snap, crackle, and pop isn't just for breakfast anymore. These noises can also be heard during a reflexology treatment. They usually can be heard or even felt when working with the joints. They are the same noises you might hear during a chiropractic adjustment.

These noises are usually caused by little air bubbles in the synovial fluid between your joints popping. When the toes or ankles are rotated or maneuvered just so, these little bubbles can be squashed and popped, hence the sound. If you're working on someone who has arthritis or a degeneration of the bones, the crunching, snapping, and popping noises could actually be the joints rubbing together. If this is the case, the person usually hears these sounds each time they walk barefoot, and usually the feet are very sore or tender to the touch. Be very careful when working with degenerative bone conditions. Always use a lighter touch with these people.

> **Tread Lightly**
>
> When working with someone with a degenerative bone condition, work lightly to avoid unintentionally breaking a weakened bone. People with osteoarthritis or osteoporosis have porous bones that are vulnerable to breaking.

Other times, you may hear crunchies, which must be the sound of the concentration of nerve fibers being broken up in the congested reflex area. Feet and hands that crack, snap, and pop can be thought of as having too much of the air element, indicated by the little air bubbles in the joints.

If you have lots of popping and cracking in all your joints—feet, hands, back, neck, and jaw—it could mean you have a trace mineral imbalance. All the minerals in the body work together to keep the body in balance. When there's a deficiency of mineral intake in the diet (a common occurrence these days with our mineral-depleted soils), it causes a mineral imbalance in the body. The body takes what it needs from our reserves of minerals in the body, such as calcium from the bones or magnesium from the muscles, to get what it needs to balance.

# Water: Puff, the Magic Ankles

When you first look at the foot and see that it's swollen in certain areas—or just plain swollen all over—ask the person if they twisted or sprained their ankle recently, which could be a cause of the swelling. Be sure, before working on someone with swollen ankles, that the swelling doesn't fall under one of the contraindication categories (see Chapter 6).

If a twist or sprain isn't the cause of the swelling, then your subject more than likely has an overabundance of the water element. This is especially true if the person also has a puffy face and fingers. You may suspect the person is holding excess water in their entire body. If this is so, it could mean sluggishness in the urinary system, the lymphatic system or, as we learned earlier, an imbalanced thyroid or other endocrine disorder. Simple lymphatic stagnation can happen when a person has been sitting or inactive all day, especially during long airplane flights. Dehydration can aggravate the condition, so please don't forget to stay hydrated by drinking plenty of pure water throughout the day.

> **Tip Toe**
>
> Water retention can mean either that the person has too much water or, ironically, that the person is on the verge of dehydration and the body is holding on to water to protect itself. Either way, the urinary and lymphatic systems need to be stimulated to help this condition.

# Work Those Lymphs!

When the ankles are swollen, be sure to work on all the lymphatic areas between the metatarsals and the lower lymph areas all across and around the ankles. The next area you should work on is the urinary system. The kidneys could be ineffective, and potassium levels could be low. Stimulate the kidney and bladder areas, and note any tenderness there.

Instead of having too much water, the body could be holding on to water because it's in a state of dehydration! When the body is consistently not getting enough water, it can have a tendency to hold on to fluids. This retention goes away after drinking enough water daily for the body to let go of its stash.

# Go with the Flow

In my experience, if someone has swollen areas on their feet when they come in for reflexology, they won't have swollen feet when they leave. Reflexology helps stimulate the lymphatic system and gets things moving again. The following can also help relieve water retention—just take them with a tall glass of water:

- ◆ B-complex vitamins
- ◆ Juniper berries
- ◆ Parsley
- ◆ Dandelion root
- ◆ Cornsilk
- ◆ Buchu root

> **Foot Note**
>
> In a group of reflexology studies compiled by the American Reflexology Certification Board, a Danish study revealed that reflexology treatments have a pain-relieving effect on acute kidney stone complaints. The study shows that 9 of 10 patients in the therapy group experienced no pain following the treatment.

# Slimy, Sweaty Feet

Sometimes you'll see a pair of profusely sweating feet. Kind of like a wet fish, these feet are difficult to hold on to. Sweaty feet are an obvious overabundance of the water element in the body. Because the pores on the feet are the largest, this is a convenient place for the body to eliminate moisture.

The body can only eliminate water for so long, though. Eventually, there's the danger of the well running dry, so to speak. Balancing the water element is definitely a necessity.

Conditions that cause excessive sweating in the feet can be linked with nervousness or a great amount of stress. When we're nervous or stressed, the body is more likely to sweat. Work on this person's nervous system and adrenal glands. Of course, the urinary system is part of the water element, so work on the bladder and kidney reflexes also.

The best way to perform reflexology on someone who has an overly wet condition of the feet is to work with a clean, absorbent cotton sock on the foot and work through it or use a terry-cloth towel over the area so you don't slip off the reflex pressure points. If this is something you're not comfortable with, you can also try applying some cornstarch or talcum powder to the feet to help dry them before working on the reflexes.

### Tip Toe

When there's too much water in the body, it requires a little bit of warmth (fire) to evaporate and balance the water. Be sure you use a lukewarm washcloth to bathe this type of feet before you start. The cloth can be somewhat dry, and adding a little golden seal powder to the cloth helps dry up and may slightly disinfect the feet before you work on them.

# Earth: Stiff Toes, Stiff Neck

Many times you'll observe a pair of feet with toes that are curled in and feel very tight or stiff. If you ask the person to spread out their toes, you'll usually still not be able to see any space between their toes.

When you try to perform tootsie rolls (see Chapter 6) on these toes, it will feel more like rolling a pencil between your fingers! On the element model, this could be considered too much earth: too much structure, stiffness, and rigidity. Earth is the hardest of all elements and the most solid.

The best therapies for these stiff, tight toes are full toe rotations, tootsie rolls, and the knuckle technique (where you push your knuckles into the padding of the ball of the foot). This opens up the toes and the spaces between and gets some circulation and flexibility back to these areas. (See Chapter 7 for a refresher on using the knuckle press technique.)

Another good way to help these toes spread out is to put your fingers between as many toes as you can while doing an ankle rotation. In a way, you're trying to get air (space) in this dense, earthy condition to break it up and spread it out.

> **Tread Lightly** _____
>
> Be very, very gentle with stiff, crackly toes, as these toes could break while you're performing reflexology! Be sure to support the toes well with your other hand as you're using your fingers to very gently rotate the toes one at a time.

# Fire: Feet That Flame On

A bright red foot is a good indication that there's an overabundance of fire in the feet. Red is the color associated with fire. There's a lot of blood going to a red area.

Excessive heat is another clue that a person has too much fire. For example, the clients I see who have arthritic feet with much pain also have very red, hot feet. There's no need to warm up my hands before working on these people. Inflammation and heat also signify an over-abundance of the fire element. Think of the word *inflame*—it actually describes fire!

Hot, red feet might signal a problem with the circulatory system. Fire, manifested as inflammation, could be caused by infection, or autoimmune diseases where the immune system is attacking the body's own tissues or joints, such as in the case of rheumatoid arthritis. The circulation to the feet or any affected area could be stagnant as well, adding to the swelling. Reflexology benefits these conditions because it helps bring better circulation to the feet, relaxes muscles and helps to balance the immune system.

Because the circulatory system falls within the fire category, you should take a look at the health of the entire circulatory system. Is it inefficient? Why is the blood going to the feet and then staying there? Is there a blockage somewhere in the veins or arteries that's inhibiting the free flow of blood, or could it be another condition such as arteriosclerosis? Does the person have hemorrhoids? Hemorrhoids are just swollen veins in an inconvenient place. Then again, if they were more convenient, what would we do with them?

### Tip Toe

To reflex the area for hemorrhoids, you should first work the entire colon, because hemorrhoids are usually caused by constipation. Then work on the reflex corresponding to the rectum, which is the area on the left foot and left palm where the colon ends—this is just below and slightly overlaps the bladder reflex.

Use reflexology with the goal of improving circulation. The techniques that stretch and maneuver the feet gently but vigorously, such as yummies and rotations of the toes and ankles, aid a person with an imbalance of fire. It helps get the fire moving to other areas. Also work the heart area on the padding of the ball of the left foot.

You don't want to add fuel to the fire, so you shouldn't attempt to keep a hot or inflamed foot wrapped up in a heating pad like you might like to do with someone with cold feet. This can only aggravate the fire condition. Reflexologists work only one foot at a time, so it's important to keep the foot that isn't being worked on comfortable. A cool approach such as gently wrapping the foot in a very soft flannel cloth does nicely, and adding a few mists of a cool peppermint or birch essential oil spray to the foot can feel wonderful to the client with too much fire in the feet. You might also gently wipe or dab their feet with a cool, wet sponge that has a little birch essential oil on it before their treatment. Not only can this help cool inflammation but working with pure essential oils always adds a nice aroma to the room.

See how you can use your understanding of the four elements in your reflexology treatments? In Chapter 19, we take a look at the personality side of the feet. You can keep the four elements in mind while you read through Chapter 19, as each element definitely has its own "personality."

## The Least You Need to Know

◆ Using the characteristics of the four elements—earth, air, water, and fire—to observe the feet, you may determine what elements are missing or overabundant and apply the most appropriate methods to encourage balance.

◆ Popping or cracking joints can indicate too much air. This is balanced by earth. Too much earth, however, can cause stiffness.

◆ Sweaty or swollen feet indicate too much of the water element. Work the lymphatic system, and use a warming and drying element for balance.

◆ Fire or hot conditions in the feet can indicate a problem with inflammation and can be soothed with cooling applications added to your reflexology session.

# Chapter 18

# Podiatry Matters

## In This Chapter

- ◆ Discover how to identify some common foot problems
- ◆ Find out how to deal with athlete's foot
- ◆ Learn about bone spurs, hammer toes, bunions, and more
- ◆ Understand the importance of wearing proper shoes
- ◆ Apply some natural remedies for some common foot conditions

By now you may have worked on everyone's feet in your family, and hopefully you've been experimenting on yourself, too! But besides all those metaphorical and philosophical ways to look at feet, how do you identify an obvious physical problem? This chapter helps you identify some of these problems and teaches how you can avoid getting yourself into any of these conditions in the first place. Now take off your shoes and follow in my footsteps …

# The Doctor Is In

Remember, a reflexologist is not a *podiatrist* (foot doctor) and should never give medical advice or diagnose conditions. However, as a reflexologist, you'll gain familiarity with many conditions of the feet.

This chapter gives you a holistic view of some common foot ailments. It also describes these ailments and their probable causes. I offer some tips throughout to help you and your friends and family members help themselves with natural remedies. Otherwise, you can refer them to a foot specialist.

## def•i•ni•tion

Podiatry is the health profession that cares for the human foot. The doctor of podiatric medicine is called a **podiatrist** and he examines, treats diseases, injuries, and defects of the foot, and gives a diagnosis.

Dr. Robert Timm, a podiatrist from Colorado and teacher of foot joint realignment and reflexology, says, "Reflexologists need to understand that not all sensitive areas are reflex points that need stimulation. It could be a local problem such as Morton's neuroma, plantar fascitis, a tumor, a plantar wart, osteochrondritis, a malpositioned joint, a cyst, arthritis, a corn, or a callus caused by a joint that is misaligned, however slightly."

It's important to understand and be able to recognize some of these local problems and know how to work with or around these ailments. I discuss in this chapter some common problems you may see and touch on a few things you shouldn't touch on!

# An Athletic Fungus

*Tinea pedis* is the medical term for a condition we all have heard of called athlete's foot. Athlete's foot is a contagious fungal condition. The term "athlete's foot" came about because it has been a common condition among athletes who share locker rooms (barefoot) and showers.

## Don't Sweat It

Symptoms of athlete's foot include itching, scaling, and even cracking of the skin. Sometimes small blisters appear. Treatment for athlete's foot varies from soaking the feet in potassium permanganate solution to

applying commercial antifungal ointments or powders. Natural remedies include the use of tea-tree oil to rid the skin of the fungus.

The best preventative medicine against athlete's foot is to wear flip-flops
in locker rooms and locker-room showers. Try to keep your feet dry, and
don't keep sweaty socks on your feet for any length of time.

Because contagious infections of the feet and hands fall under the contraindications chart for reflexology, you need to know how to identify
them and should politely decline to work on a person with an infection.
Don't assume the person will tell you they have this condition when
they make an appointment with you. Many times people are unaware
it's a problem and don't even know it's contagious!

# Bone Spurs and Other Missteps

A person is usually very aware of a bone spur—a sharp projection of
bone—when they have one. These are usually caused because calcium is
out of solution in the body. This is nutritionally caused by a trace mineral deficiency.

Bone spurs are easy to identify by observing the foot. They can be seen
as little, hard bumps protruding from the foot or hand and can be as
large as a marble. They usually occur around the wrists or the heel of
the foot.

When you see a bone spur, don't get spurred on to work on it! Some
people have been known to smash their own bone spurs against a hard
surface, breaking them up to be eliminated or reabsorbed by the body
naturally afterward. I wouldn't suggest you do this to anyone. When
a bone spur is present, do not work directly on the bone spur. Work
around the area.

**Tip Toe**

Hydrangea is an herb used historically to dissolve calculus buildup
and stones in the body such as kidney stones, bladder stones, and
bone spurs. Hydrangea may be swallowed and usually comes in
capsules. Some have applied the essential oil of birch to these areas
and have claimed the spurs have disappeared with regular use in a
matter of weeks.

## Tool Time for Hammer Toes

*Hammer toe* is a deformity of a toe. Most often this occurs in the second toe (also known as the wealth toe) and is caused by fixed flexion of the first joint. In other words, the joint of the toe gets permanently fixed in a bent position and cannot be straightened.

Hammer toe can be very painful, and usually (because most of us have to wear shoes every day) the pressure from a shoe on top of a hammer toe or toes causes friction and can create a callus or corn on top of the toe. This makes it even more hardened and painful.

> **def•i•ni•tion**
>
> **Hammer toe** is an actual deformity of a toe caused by fixed flexion of the first joint. The joint gets permanently fixed in a bent position.

When working on someone with a hammer toe or toes, flexibility will be an issue. Try to get the person to loosen up and work especially with techniques that stretch and rotate the feet. Do not work directly on top of the hammer toe or corn that might have developed there.

Don't try to force these toes to straighten out! This could be very painful for the subject. Now, over time, if the person wears proper-fitting shoes and comes for reflexology regularly, this condition may just work itself out. The problem is that the tightness in the muscles is keeping the toe in a bent position. Therefore, work on loosening the muscles around the metatarsals. But use extreme caution to avoid forcing the toes or hurting an individual with this condition. Toe rotations are also good to use on those with hammer toes.

## Not-So-Golden Arches

Some folks have what is called *fallen arches*. The arches in their feet have actually fallen, which can be a very painful condition. Many times, there is a lack of muscle tone in the entire body when you see this condition. Those who gain a large amount of weight in a short period of time often suffer from fallen arches.

When the arches fall, there could be torn ligaments or strained muscles in the bottom of the foot. Be gentle on folks with this problem. If you have fallen arches, try the following:

◆ Get some exercise.

◆ Walk barefoot in the sand.

◆ Use a foot roller daily.

◆ Use your toes to pick up small objects such as marbles or small rubber balls.

**def•i•ni•tion**

**Fallen arches** can happen with prolonged standing or excessive weight, tearing or weakening the muscles of the arch and causing flat feet.

Sometimes orthotics prescribed by a podiatrist or even a chiropractor help the person regain support.

# When Good Women Love Bad Shoes

If the shoe fits, wear it. Literally, this should be a rule for all of us. Most of us wear ill-fitting shoes that cause corns, calluses, and deformation of the bones of the feet. Remember how much weight our feet bear. We need to wear good shoes to allow our feet to walk correctly and support us as we walk through life.

You've probably guessed that the females of the species are the ones most guilty of choosing shoes for looks and style over pure comfort. I am personally guilty of jamming my feet into all sorts of shoes as a young girl to hide my size 8½ flippers!

Be sure you pick shoes that have a wide enough toe box for the width of your feet. If not, the weight of the foot, especially when there's a lift or incline on the shoe, pushes the weight up to the ball of the foot. Then the toes are jammed together tightly into the toe box. This causes deformities such as hammer toes or bunions.

Many times these conditions require surgery, so work first on prevention. What would you do if you had to walk a mile in your own shoes? Think about that before you purchase your next pair.

# This Little Piggy Had Corn

Little piggies may like corn, but your feet's little piggies think they are a painful nuisance. The medical term for a corn is a *keratosis*. A keratosis is any horny growth of the skin. The keratosis is caused by constant pressure or repeated friction on a toe. Corns are raised, circular lumps

**def•i•ni•tion**

> Keratosis is any horny growth of the skin. The most common ones are warts and corns.

that are usually yellow and resemble a kernel of corn, hence the name. The base of the corn is at the surface, and the tip lies in the deeper tissue of the skin. Sometimes the corn is even attached to bone!

Many times, corns need to be surgically removed. The cause, again, is ill-fitting shoes. So wear proper shoes—I can't emphasize that enough.

When you're working on someone with corns, do not work directly on the corn itself, as it may cause pain to the bone it's attached to.

## Painful Plantar Warts

Plantar warts are another problem and are normally caused by virus. The roots of a plantar wart can run deep into the foot, so don't work directly on a plantar wart, as it can be painful.

**Tip Toe**

A plantar wart is caused by a virus in the body. Some reflexologists link the location of a plantar wart on the foot to a virus in the part of the body the wart corresponds to. This is probably a stretch, but nonetheless a concept it couldn't hurt to check out!

## Do You Cry When You Peel a Bunion?

*Bunions* are another bone deformation of the foot. A bunion occurs when the big toe overlaps another toe. This condition sometimes results from a heredity trait called *hallux valgus*, although an improper-fitting shoe can also cause the problem.

**def•i•ni•tion**

> *Hallux valgus* is a deviation of the big toe at its metatarsophalangeal joint. This deviation causes what is known as a **bunion**. *Hallux* is Latin for "great toe," and *valgus* means "an overt positional deformity, turning away from the midline of the body."

*Hallux valgus* is a deviation of the big toe at its metatarsophalangeal joint. As a result, the bursa is enlarged, and because it's an area often affected by constant rubbing, a callus develops over the area, which forms the bunion.

Bunions are more likely to occur in women than men. Tight shoes with high heels and pointed toes are likely to cause this condition. Commercially available felt pads can help relieve the pressure. If the bunion is extremely painful, a surgical procedure to realign the phalanges and remove excess bone tissue may be performed.

Do not push directly on a bunion. Bunions most commonly occur around the thyroid reflex area. Work the inside of the thyroid area, and be gentler on the outside where the bunion is. Never try to force a toe back to its proper position. Be aware of the bunion and work around it, especially if it is inflamed.

> **Tread Lightly**
>
> Never work directly on any bone disorders of the feet such as bunions or hammer toes. Also, do not push directly on bone spurs, corns, or plantar warts.

## Grows (in) on You

Ill-fitting shoes can also cause ingrown toenails. An ingrown toenail is a condition in which the sharp end of a toenail grows into the flesh of a toe. It's most common on the big toe. The tissue around the toenail may become infected, causing discomfort. Trimming the toenails improperly can also cause ingrown toenails. Toenails should be cut straight across when trimming.

Because there is already pressure causing pain to the toe with an ingrown nail, do not apply any pressure to this toe when performing reflexology!

# Some Natural Remedies

Obviously, proper care of your feet is very important; after all, your feet carry you where you want to go. Wearing proper-fitting shoes and simple precautions can prevent most of the problems highlighted in this chapter.

When your feet hurt, you hurt all over, and it lowers your stamina and your spirits. Try reflexology as a natural healing therapy, and consider some other natural remedies listed in the following table.

# Natural Remedies for Common Foot Ailments

| Condition | Natural Remedies | Reflexology Tips |
|---|---|---|
| Athlete's foot | Tea-tree oil applied one to two times a day directly to infected area (entire foot or hand), morning and night. When condition dries up and clears, golden seal added to a bit of honey and beeswax makes a nice foot balm or salve. Prevent future infection by wearing flip-flops in community showers/locker rooms, and keep feet dry when possible. | Reflex all lympathic system reflexes and immune system components. |
| Stinky feet | Zinc—up to 45mg per day for the average adult. Remember, if you stink, take zinc. Pumpkin seeds or encapsulated herbs commonly labeled as herbal pumpkin also contain a good amount of a natural form of zinc, which may prove helpful. Liquid chlorophyll added to water daily also helps deodorize the entire body. An activated charcoal supplement should be useful as well. | Work on the reflexes to the kidneys. Imbalances in the kidneys cause odorous feet. Work the reflexes to the whole urinary system, reproductive system, lymphatics, and all endocrine glands. |
| Plantar warts | Footbaths. Place both feet in very hot water and then very cold water. Alternate until hot water cools. *Do not try this if you have a weakened heart or high blood pressure*—the increase in circulation | Work lymphatics, immune, and liver reflexes. |

| Condition | Natural Remedies | Reflexology Tips |
|---|---|---|
| | could cause problems. A teaspoon of colloidal (liquid) silver taken internally for 10 days may help kill viruses. Silver is a trace mineral that can be found at most health food stores or through herbal or other natural supplement distributors. It should be used only temporarily. Tea-tree oil applied topically to warts after each footbath should prove helpful. The warts should be gone in a week or so. | |
| Bone spurs | Usually occur because calcium is out of solution in the body, caused by a mineral imbalance. Supplement with a good herbal calcium and a multi-mineral supplement such as colloidal minerals or alfalfa. Hydrangea has been used historically to break up calcium deposits. Take until spur disappears and then continue supplementing with alfalfa or another natural mineral supplement. | Work parathyroid reflexes, heart, and small intestines. |
| Fallen arches | Foot exercises such as picking up small items with the toes, orthotics, and a weight-loss program. | Work the heart, small intestine, and kidney reflexes. |

I hope using these natural remedies can save you or a loved one an unnecessary trip to the doctor—and you've learned a way to help your feet and help yourself!

## The Least You Need to Know

◆ Athlete's foot is a contagious fungal infection of the skin of the feet. When you see this condition on someone you want to work on, please reschedule the reflexology after the infection clears.

◆ Never work directly on a bone spur, corn, or ingrown toenail, as this will cause pain.

◆ One of the most important things you can do to avoid foot dysfunction is to wear proper-fitting shoes.

◆ Tea-tree oil has been used to clear up fungal conditions of the skin.

◆ If your feet stink, take zinc! But don't overdo it, about 45 mg per day is max.

# 19

# The Personality in the Feet

## In This Chapter

- ◆ See how your feet can show the path you've walked in life
- ◆ Learn to recognize more elemental conditions of the feet
- ◆ Discover what the lines on your feet say about you
- ◆ Find some indicators of wealth on the hands and feet
- ◆ See what your moles and freckles may be telling you

Our feet carry us through life, and by observing their physical shape and condition, we can gain insight into how we walk through life. Do we skip merrily or just shuffle along? Have we traveled a "hard road," or have we floated or even been carried through life?

In this chapter, we take a peek at what the condition, shape, and signs on the feet and hands might reveal about the way we walk the earth, the way we think, and maybe even the lessons we need to learn. What type of footprints do you want to leave behind?

# High-Arched and Up in the Clouds

Do you walk on your toes? Do you like to tiptoe through the tulips? Do you have high arches? In foot personality analysis, a person with high arches is a dreamer, inventor, thinker, and one who has his head in the clouds! (High arches would fall into the air category on the four-element chart—see Chapter 17.)

The high arches keep a person up in the air. People with high arches usually like to travel, especially by air. People with their heads in the clouds can think up things that some of us cannot fathom. They are visionaries who make great consultants to companies who want to see the "big picture." These people can help us get prepared for the future through their ability to see beyond today. Sometimes they are ahead of their time.

## High Achievers

People with high arches many times have high ideals and high expectations of themselves and others. They are forward thinkers and actively take part in life. Living in the clouds makes it easier for high-arched people to change directions quickly and easily, and our high-arched friends can confuse us at times when they quickly switch directions.

> **Tip Toe**
>
> If a high-arched partner comes bouncing into your life, get ready for some stimulating intellectual conversations while you're packing your bags for the trip you'll be going on together. The high-arched of the world love to travel!

High-arched folks spend much of their time up in the air, where there are no landmarks. The high-arched person feels free and unencumbered because of this, but it can drive the more grounded, earthy people a little crazy! Many people with high arches work in the computer industry, an intellectually dominated, forward-thinking, technology-driven market.

## Walking on Air

High-arched people enjoy flight and many become pilots, hang gliders, and skydivers. They can't get enough of taking their feet off the ground! Usually, these folks walk with a bounce in their step and are not as concerned about the mundane matters of life. They are more focused on ideals and creativity.

They can be natural experts in engineering design, because they can see how everything fits together in the grand scheme of things. But they probably won't want to work physically building the pieces.

Reflexology is a great therapy for folks with high arches because it tends to "bring them back down to Earth" and can be very grounding and comforting to those who are intellectually driven. Reflexology can help these people get more in touch with their bodies.

# Flat-Footed and Down to Earth

The opposite of high arches is flat feet, which are feet with no arches at all. In contrast to the high-arched folks, flat-footed folks are more grounded. People with flat feet feel a real connection to the earth. They enjoy being in the forest, out in nature, and like the feeling of their feet on the ground. People with flat feet can enjoy reflexology because they're in tune with the physical pleasures of the body—more so than the high-arched folks.

Sometimes flat-footed people have a feeling of being unsupported. These people can feel as if they're carrying more responsibility on their life path. Flat-footed people may feel a drive to achieve and may be overburdened with this responsibility.

## Earth Mothers

Having such a strong connection to the earth, many times flat-footed people work with earth-oriented organizations, protecting the rights of indigenous peoples or working to protect the environment.

Flat-footed people need to be careful not to become martyrs and should sometimes let themselves break free of their self-induced burdens. A good reflexology treatment utilizing uplifting aromatherapy oils, such as a mixture of bergamot and pink grapefruit on the temples, is an excellent therapy for the flat-footed person.

---

**Foot Note**

Although flat-footed folks enjoy music that's earthier, such as Indian flute music, they should be encouraged to listen to harp or piano music once in a while. Music by Bach or Mozart falls more in the air element and helps disconnect a flat-footed person from his worries over the plight of the earth and its inhabitants.

---

## What Makes Your Toes Curl?

In Chapter 17, I talked about the stiff toes/stiff neck scenario in the feet. But other than too much of the earth element or tight toe boxes squashing the toes together, why do people hold their toes curled under? In a word: *fear.*

Because the toes represent the head area, curling the toes under is a subconscious protective position. It can be like hiding your head in the sand or covering your face. On a day-to-day level, when you're unsure about something, fearful, or not ready yet to face the music, so to speak, you might be curling up your toes to "lessen the impact" of what you're hearing or seeing. Curled toes can also be a metaphor for gripping or hanging on to persons, things, or events too tightly. The need to trust and let go is key for those with curled toes.

So the next time you're sitting with your shoes off and watching a scary movie, or listening to someone on the phone talk about something you are afraid to hear, take notice if your toes are curled under. If they are, relax—to face our fears is to grow! Then uncurl those toes and ask your hubby to work your adrenal reflexes!

# The Callused Personality

A callused *sole* doesn't necessarily mean a callused *soul*, but it could indicate a callused personality! *Calluses* are common on the foot. They occur naturally the more a person walks barefoot or wears ill-fitting shoes.

A real callus is thick skin on the foot caused by constant friction or pressure on the area. In life, when we're exposed to constant struggles, abusive situations, and irritations, we can become callused or hardened to those situations or emotions.

**def•i•ni•tion**

A **callus** is a thickened portion of the epidermal layer of the skin. Repeated friction or constant pressure to the foot or hands causes calluses.

Calluses on the skin or in our personality are meant to protect us from the outside influences that hurt us. Someone who had a hard life but has become stronger in spite of it may have callused feet. Calluses are not just the body's way of toughening up, but metaphorically are the personality's way of toughening up those areas of our lives that have been abused.

---

### Foot Note

More than likely, when you meet a person with extremely callused feet, they'll be crunchy on the outside but soft in the middle. People who have been through great pain in their lives are usually the people with the greatest character and strength and also the deepest compassion for others. When you get past the callused layer in the personality, you'll find that these people have hearts of gold.

---

To deal with calluses on the feet, administer footbaths with Epsom salts added to the water to help loosen the dead skin layers. Then use a pumice stone or some other abrasive material to remove the calluses. If you're giving reflexology to a very callused foot, you might want to have your subject soak their feet in a footbath first, or consider a wax dip, which softens the feet before a session.

See where your calluses are, and think about them in terms of the areas of the body they reflect. Do you have a callus on your large toe, representing the head area? Did you experience a great amount of verbal or mental abuse in your past? Does your heart area have a callus? How does this relate to your affairs of the heart? The heel represents your lower body or reproductive areas. Could issues over children or not having children, contribute to a callus on the heel? Think about these things, deal with the issues, and then pumice those suckers away!

# Filled with Emotion: Swollen Feet

Physically, a very swollen foot and ankle can indicate edema or lymphatic congestion. But what if the feet and ankles have always been, and still are, puffy? This usually indicates that a person holds water easily. Proper minerals, exercise, ample water intake, and reflexology should correct this problem, but swollen feet can also have an emotional connection.

In the four-element table (see Chapter 17), water relates to emotion. Holding on to water could indicate that a person has a hard time expressing emotions and is holding on to them. This person needs to learn to release repressed emotions, to let things flow and roll off their back, and not take everything personally or so deeply. This is easier said than done, but it's a good growing experience for the person with water-retentive feet.

The person who retains water/emotion has a tendency to brood or be hurt deeply by things people say or do to them, even when others' intentions were not to hurt them. Water retainers can cry easily or hold on to hurt or depression for long periods of time.

**Tip Toe**

The water-retentive person should try to come up for air sometimes, take things a little more lightheartedly, and work to prevent water retention to help with their emotions. Sometimes, retaining water can put pressure on the brain and make us feel more vulnerable, sensitive, and emotional, as with PMS. Minerals, water, B-complex vitamins, and reflexology can all help release excess water.

# Hot or Cold, Wet or Dry?

Hot feet indicate an excess of the fire element. People who have warm hands and feet are usually warm all over. They can be considered hot-tempered, hot-headed, or thought to have a very warm heart. Hot feet, of course, can indicate painful conditions of the feet, but here we are addressing the fiery type of condition in the personality.

Usually, hot feet can mean a person is very passionate. He or she may love romance. These people can get fiercely angry, but usually the anger is gone as soon as they're done expressing themselves. Hot feet usually belong to willful people. Heat comes from the blood. The blood is near the surface in those with hot extremities.

The fire energy in these people usually runs on the surface. They may wear their hearts on their sleeve, so to speak, and be influenced very easily by a "pretty face" that appeals to their sexual or romantic inclinations. Stamina may be short-lived, however. They are fast to ignite a creative idea or plans and also like the idea of making a fast buck. Hot feet can mean impatience.

Remember that if a hot-footed hot-head ever gets angry with you, they will forget about it shortly after they express it! Don't hold on to this scolding—especially if you're a water-retentive person! Let it go, because more than likely, the hot-foot has already forgotten about it!

## Cold Feet Run Deep

Cold feet and hands can indicate a person who keeps their emotions on the inside. They are not as expressive with their feelings as a hot-footed person. They can have more poise and remain calm and controlled even in emergency situations.

The cold-footed person has deep-running emotions. This can make them more insightful and self-reflective than those who immediately

> **Tread Lightly**
>
> Cold feet can mean slow circulation or metabolism. Consider anemia or low thyroid activity. Be sure to keep the feet warm and offer your subject a blanket. Cold feet can lower the body temperature and make someone feel cold all over.

express their thoughts. *Introspective* is a good word for chronically cold-handed and -footed folks. On the physical level, check for an underfunctioning thyroid or anemia if the body, hands, and feet are chronically cold and fatigued.

## Never Let Them See You Sweat

Water relates to our emotions, and releasing too much water, in a metaphorical sense, may mean a person is not sensitive to life issues. They let their emotions "run out at the bottom" and, therefore, life is not too meaningful. They may be out of touch with the deeper meanings of life.

They can also be people who have had trouble in the past having their emotions validated and, therefore, are nervous about what they feel is proper. Sweaty feet can belong to nervous folks who have a need to share their emotions but feel they cannot. This leaves them at odds with what they really want to express and what they fear they may lose by this expression. Chronically sweaty feet could be a person's discreet way of letting out their emotions without having to express or intellectualize these feelings.

**Tip Toe**

If you have a very dry or scaly foot, check for dehydration or any problems with the urinary system. Dry-footed people could have a dry sense of humor and tend toward dry conditions such as itchy, dry, flaky skin, dandruff, psoriasis, sneezing, and nervous system conditions. Dry feet fall into the air category on the four-element model (see Chapter 17).

# Footloose

Loose feet that are overly flexible and lacking in tone can indicate very open, flexible people who go with the flow of life. Sometimes they are blamed for being unorganized because they lack any form of rigidity and structure. Some amount of structure is required for organization.

These people may not show up on time for appointments, which doesn't really bother them. Type B personalities are usually the owners of very flexible feet. They are easy to get along with because they usually take things in stride, but don't expect them to meet you on time!

A loose-footed person may have a hard time taking a strong stand on issues. These people can get along with others very well. Flaccid feet fall into the water and air categories on the four-element chart.

Water and air take on the shape of their containers. These people need to be aware of ill-intentioned people who may manipulate them. Loose feet can be a sign of being too lax about life and affairs and can show the need for more discipline in thoughts and ideas and discernment in judgment of people who have an influence in their lives.

# What a Stiff

On the opposite side of the coin, a foot that is stiff and rigid and has a hard time loosening up may have a personality to match! Rigid feet can mean rigidity or very structured thinking. These people can have a hard time "letting loose" and can probably really use a good reflexology session—along with a good laugh.

Such people tend to be very pragmatic, stable, and solid, which makes them just the kind of folks you would want to handle your accounting and do your taxes. These people usually have strict schedules and regimens and are always on time, if not early. These are people who are very reliable, but also not ones to take many things lightly.

On the negative side, these people lack the ability to let things fall though the cracks. They can become too set in their ways and, therefore, miss out on experiences that would expand their minds or enhance their enjoyment of life. Everyone needs to have some fun and loosen up once in a while. Work on getting to these people's sense of humor and help them relax—but be sure to keep your appointments with them and be on time!

# The Future in Your Feet and Hands

Chinese doctors, palm readers, personologists, and others have interpreted lines or crevices in the skin for years for clues to health and personality. Some can read the lines on your feet to assess your health.

This book does not go in depth into this subject, but I have included some of these interpretations here just for fun.

These ideas are based on the premise that the lines in the feet and hands are usually caused by mental or nervous tension in the body. When we're nervous, many times we wring our hands; when we're angry, we clench our fists. We're usually much less conscious of what our feet are doing, but they, too, react in response to our emotions.

In my reflexology work, the most significant lines on the feet I look for are any lines along the spinal column reflex—along the arch of the foot. When there are many lines running across this, it could indicate central nervous system tension, stress, and mental strain.

Usually, a person with many of these fine, short vertical lines has a personality that changes easily. One moment they can be high spirited, and at another moment they are feeling blue. Usually, these people are very dynamic, and when they're feeling well, they push themselves to the limits and run themselves down very quickly. A person with many lines up and down their spinal reflexes needs to find balance.

## A Fortune at Your Fingertips

Looking for money? Here are some fun things to look for:

◆ Lines that wrap completely around the wrists can be called "bracelets of wealth." They are found more on women than men. Maybe women really do control all the money! The more bracelets, the more wealth!

◆ The second toe is considered the wealth toe. If a second toe is longer than the large toe, this can indicate there is wealth in the person's future. Some believe this is the toe of intelligence. Many times, intelligence and money go hand in hand.

◆ Look for a large M on the palm of your hand. This can mean good luck in money or in marriage—or both!

◆ Curl your hand up into a fist with your fingertips facing toward you. Look for the pointy fold sticking out the side of your hand just below the pinky joint. This is called your pocketbook. If the skin is thick and full, this could indicate that your money purse will be filled up and bulging with money!

I've seen a lot of lines in my days as a reflexologist, and you'd be surprised at how often these prove to be true.

## Jin Shin Jyutsu

Jin Shin Jyutsu is an ancient art passed down from generation to generation by word of mouth until it was revived in the early 1900s by Master Jiro Murai in Japan, who used only this energy work to clear himself of a life-threatening illness. This knowledge was handed down to Mary Burmeister, who brought it to the United States in the 1950s.

In Jin Shin Jyutsu, each finger represents an emotion and also two major organ energy patterns. The emotions and energy patterns associated with each finger are laid out in the following table.

| Finger | Related Emotion | Left Side Organ | Right Side Organ | Related Element |
|---|---|---|---|---|
| Thumb | Worry | Stomach | Spleen | Earth |
| Pointer finger | Fear | Bladder | Kidney | Water |
| Middle finger | Anger | Gallbladder | Liver | Earth (or wood) |
| Ring finger | Sadness | Large intestine | Lung | Air |
| Pinky finger | Try to/ pretense | Small intestine | Heart | Fire |

A good way to remember the emotions associated with your fingers is to remember a memory aid my teacher Isabelle Hutton, R.N., taught me: "Get rid of Worry F.A.S.T.!" Starting with the thumb, which is Worry, then the pointer finger Fear, middle finger Anger, ring finger Sadness, and the pinky, Trying to (or pretense).

## Say It with Freckles: Larry, Curly, and Mole

Moles and freckles are just a concentration of pigment on the skin. Energetically, a concentration of pigment is a concentration of energy in the body. Therefore, some believe that anywhere a mole or freckle is found on the feet or hands indicates a concentration of energy in the corresponding body part, which is density (excess earth) in that area.

If you find moles or freckles on your feet or hands, consider the reflex point you find them on. This can be a sign of a genetically inherited congestion in the corresponding area. You might want to consider an internal cleansing program designed to cleanse that particular organ. The moles or freckles won't usually disappear, but you might want to do something that will decongest the particular part, just for preventative medicine's sake.

For example, if you find a freckle on the ball of your foot and also one on the top of your foot, you might think about your lung and chest area. There may be a concentration of energy there. You can work preventatively on yourself by avoiding living in a heavily polluted environment and staying away from smoking. Because the freckle is also on the chest reflex, if you're a woman, be sure you visit your doctor regularly for mammograms. Most important, use reflexology to rub out those tender areas in the corresponding reflex areas (in this case, the lung and upper chest).

---

**Tip Toe**

I had a client who had a large freckle on her left ovary reflex on the heel. Just to test the validity of the idea that moles or freckles can indicate a genetically inherited condition, I asked her if her mother had any type of female problems. She said her mom died of ovarian cancer!

---

**Foot Note**

One of my massage therapists told me that a freckle on the bottom of my foot meant I was condemned as a witch in a past life and burned at the stake! I wonder if my freckle was the last ash that was left. (Don't *ash* me, I'm just the reflexologist.)

My husband has a freckle on the bottom of his foot in exactly the same place as I do. We take this coincidence to mean we are soulmates and meant to be together. Either that or he was a warlock who charred along with me! How's that for a smokin' relationship?

## The Least You Need to Know

◆ High arches can mean a person is intellectually driven. Reflexology treatments can help this person come down to Earth.

◆ Flat feet can mean a person feels heavy with responsibility and unsupported. Help this person melt away their burdens with reflexology.

◆ Calluses on the feet can mean a person has had much adversity in life and has built up resistance, but they are usually soft at heart.

◆ Rigid feet can mean a rigid personality. Help the person loosen up with reflexology.

◆ Freckles or moles can indicate a concentration of energy in the corresponding body part.

# What Does It All Mean? A Brief Glossary

**acupressure**   A traditional Chinese therapeutic technique whereby pressure is applied to acupuncture points. Acupuncture and acupressure use the same points; the difference is that acupuncture utilizes sterile needles, and acupressure does not penetrate the skin.

**alveoli**   Small pockets that stick out along the walls of alveolar sacs in the lung. This is where carbon dioxide leaves the blood and the blood takes in oxygen.

**aromatherapy**   The therapeutic use of aroma or smells to gain a positive, desired effect.

**asthma**   A condition characterized by attacks of bronchospasms causing difficulty in breathing. Asthma is brought on by an array of stimuli, including allergens, exertion, emotions, and infections.

**athlete's foot**   A contagious fungal condition similar to ringworm. The medical name for this infection is *tinea pedis*. Athlete's foot was so named because it's a common condition among athletes who share locker rooms (barefoot) and showers.

**bedside manner**   A term used to describe how a doctor behaves in front of or toward his patients. Reflexologists also need to develop a good bedside manner for the recipient to feel comfortable, at ease, relaxed, and well cared for.

**bipolar disorder**   A severe mental illness characterized by severe depression followed by bouts of mania. Mania takes the form of obsession, compulsion, or an exaggerated feeling of euphoria.

**body reflexology**   Similar to foot and hand reflexology but the reflexes are found over the entire body, not just on the feet and hands.

**bronchiole** A small airway of the breathing system from the bronchi to the lobes of the lung. The bronchioles allow the exchange of air and waste gases between the alveolar ducts and the bronchi.

**bronchitis** Inflammation of the bronchi. It's an illness characterized by coughing, a constriction of the bronchi due to spasms, and the production of copious amounts of mucus from the bronchi.

**central nervous system** Includes the brain and spinal cord and controls conscious thoughts and actions such as movement and talking.

**contraindication** A term meaning any factor in a condition that makes it unwise to pursue a certain line of treatment. For example, you would not give a massage to a person with severe sunburn!

**dehydration** The lack of water in body tissues. Lack of efficient water intake, vomiting, diarrhea, and sweating can all be causes of dehydration. Symptoms may include great thirst, nausea, and exhaustion. If drinking plenty of water does not immediately correct the problem, sometimes water and salts need to be administered intravenously at an emergency room.

**diabetes mellitus** A disorder of carbohydrate metabolism in which sugars in the body are not oxidized to produce energy due to lack of the pancreatic hormone insulin or to resistance to insulin. The accumulation of sugar leads to its appearance in the blood (hyperglycemia) and then in the urine. Symptoms include thirst, loss of weight, and the excessive production of urine. Complications can include poor circulation leading to slow healing, poor eyesight, weight gain, and coma if insulin and diet are not regulated. *See also* hyperglycemia.

**diverticulitis** A disease of the bowel in which compacted fecal matter causes pressure in the bowel that produces small pouches or bowel pockets along the intestinal walls. These sacs can fester and swell, causing severe discomfort. These infected pockets can be dangerous or deadly if they burst.

**endorphins** Substances in the nervous system released by the pituitary gland that affect the central nervous system by reducing pain. Their effect on the body is similar to the effects of using pain-killing medications such as morphine.

**fallen arches** Literally flat feet, caused by prolonged standing or excessive weight, tearing, or weakening of the muscles in the arches of the feet.

**femur, tibia** and **fibula,** and **patella**   All bones of the leg. The patella is the kneecap, the femur is the largest leg bone, and the tibia and fibula make up the shins.

**footbath**   The use of water and sometimes essential oils applied to the feet and lower legs to change the condition of or circulation in the body.

**four-element model**   Used as a tool to teach a philosophical way of seeing the elements (air, fire, water, and earth) in everything we do.

**gallstone**   A hard, stonelike mass made of cholesterol (blood fat), bile pigments, and calcium salts. Gallstones can cause trouble when and if they get stuck in a bile duct, where they can cause jaundice.

**glandular system**   A general term used to describe all the glands of the body. The glandular system is divided into two categories: the endocrine glands (without ducts) and exocrine glands (with ducts). Glands are considered an organ or group of cells that make and secrete fluids, such as hormones.

**goiter**   An enlargement of the thyroid gland. Goiter is usually caused by a lack of iodine. The thyroid is actually working hard to attract the nutrient iodine (its main source of food) and enlarges in the process.

***hallux valgus***   A deviation of the large toe at its metatarsophalangeal joint. This deviation causes what is known as a bunion. *Hallux* is Latin for "great toe," and *valgus* means "an overt positional deformity, turning away from the midline of the body."

**hammer toe**   A deformity of the toe. Most often this occurs in the second toe (the wealth toe!) and is caused by fixed flexion of the first joint. In other words, the joint of the toe gets permanently fixed in a bent position.

**holistic**   A term used to describe a way of living, practicing, or thinking that takes into account all factors of life. In holistic health, a practitioner considers the physical, mental, emotional, and spiritual aspects of the person to help them back to balance.

**homeostasis**   The medical term used for the body's internal balancing act. It means our unconscious body functions, such as body temperature and glandular secretions, are working for us to keep us alive and functioning. Life truly is a balancing act.

**hyperglycemia**   Also known as diabetes, a disease relating to the pancreas and its insufficient production of insulin to keep the blood sugar level balanced. Diabetes, in effect, is high blood sugar. *See also* diabetes mellitus.

**hyperthyroid**   An overactive thyroid leading to symptoms such as nervous irritability, excitability, ferocious appetite, inability to gain weight, a racing heart, and popping eyes.

**hypothyroid**   A thyroid that is worn out and underactive. It usually is too weak to produce the correct thyroid hormones. Symptoms of hypothyroidism are a general slowing down of the metabolism, causing coldness, slowed speech, slower movements, lethargy, and trouble staying asleep.

**hysterectomy**   The removal of a woman's uterus. Sometimes a full utero-ovarian hysterectomy is performed, which also removes one or both of the ovaries.

**insomnia**   The inability to fall asleep or to remain asleep for an adequate length of time.

**keratosis**   Any horny growth of the skin, most commonly seen as warts or corns.

**menopause**   When a woman's ovaries stop producing eggs. The ovaries discontinue their hormone production, which sometimes leads to dry skin, emotional instability, hot flashes, and heart palpitations.

**meridians**   Invisible lines of energy that run longitudinally along the body. The mapping of these meridian lines along the body is known as zone therapy, which many say is just another name for reflexology.

**mouse shoulder**   A spasm of the muscles behind the shoulder blade that can pull the vertebrae in the upper neck and back out of alignment. This situation is usually found on the side of the body that is used to operate a computer mouse and can cause pain and stiffness or even numbness in the arm and hand on that side.

**orthotic inserts**   Special prescription shoe inserts designed to support or supplement weakened joints or limbs.

**ovulation**   The time in a woman's menstrual cycle when the ovaries produce an egg and deliver the egg to the uterus to be (sometimes) fertilized. This process is controlled by the hormones secreted by the pituitary gland.

**PMS (premenstrual syndrome)**   A syndrome occurring in the days before menstruation. PMS symptoms may include tension, irritability, emotional disturbance, headache, abdominal bloating, tender and swollen breasts, pimples, and water retention.

**podiatry**  The health profession that cares for the human foot. The doctor of podiatric medicine is called a *podiatrist* and examines, diagnoses, and treats diseases, injuries, and defects of the foot.

**pronate** *(v.)* or **pronation** *(n.)*  The lowering of the inner edge of the foot by turning it.

**reflexology**  Literally the study of how one part reflects or relates to another part of the body. Reflexology is a holistic therapy used for health management and maintenance and can also be used as a health and personality analysis tool.

**rosacea**  A skin disease on the face in which the blood vessels on the cheeks and nose enlarge, causing the face to appear bright red or flushed. The cause is uncertain, but it's believed that extremes in temperature, food irritants, and too much alcohol all play a part in aggravating the condition.

**seasonal affective disorder (SAD)**  A syndrome characterized by severe depression during certain times of the year. This disorder brings on a desire to overeat, especially carbohydrates. Most notably the depression is experienced during times when there's a lack of sunshine. Stimulating the pineal gland may help relieve symptoms.

**sinusitis**  An inflammation of one or more of the mucus-lined air spaces in the facial bones that communicate with the nose. It's often caused by infections spreading from the nose, and symptoms include headache and tenderness over the affected sinus, which may become filled with a purulent material that's discharged through the nose.

**solar plexus**  Found right in the middle of where the rib cage comes together about at the stomach level in front of the diaphragm.

**subluxation**  An out-of-alignment joint. If you visit a chiropractor, he or she will usually diagnose you with one or more subluxations along your spinal column. Reflexology can help chiropractic adjustments last longer by keeping the muscles relaxed.

**supination**  A condition in which the foot is turned inward so the medial (outer) margin is elevated.

**symbology** or **symbolism**  Describes how a symbol can represent something else. For instance, each country has a flag that symbolizes that particular country. Everyone has their own personalized set of symbolic meanings based on their life experiences. This is why you can be the best interpreter of your own dream details.

**tinnitus** A condition characterized by any noise, buzzing, or ringing in the ear. Causes of tinnitus may be excess ear wax, damage to the eardrum, Meniere's disease, or thinning blood due to overuse of aspirin or other drugs. Dr. Bernard Jensen also links tinnitus to a lack of magnesium.

**torque** A turning or twisting force. In reflexology treatments, you need to be careful not to torque the knee, because that joint is only designed to bend one way.

**zone therapy** A term used interchangeably with reflexology. Zone therapy was coined by a medical doctor in the late 1800s and is used to describe the theory of energy zones that run longitudinally along the body.

# Index

# I

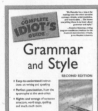
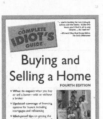
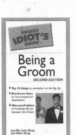
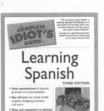

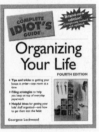
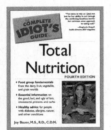
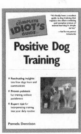
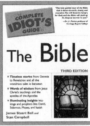
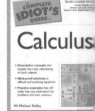
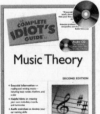
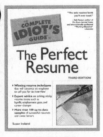
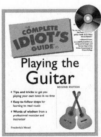
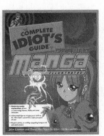
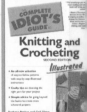